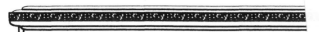

Karen Karmel-Ross
Editor

Torticollis: Differential Diagnosis, Assessment and Treatment, Surgical Management and Bracing

Pre-Publication REVIEWS, COMMENTARIES, EVALUATIONS . . .

"**T**his authoritative and up-to-date text is thorough and comprehensive and well organized. It presents helpful general guidelines and expands into etiology, extensive review of literature of conservative management/indications, assessment–including anticipated outcomes, surgical management–including history of surgical management and role of operative technique and then splinting as a conservative method of intervention or as it is used post-operatively. Postural development of the infant and child is discussed in the closing chapter.

This text will be extremely useful for the orthopaedic surgeon, pediatric surgeon, physical therapist/occupational therapist, parents and for families and others involved in the care of the child with torticollis."

John F. Sarwark, MD
Acting Division Head, Pediatric Orthopaedic Surgery, Children's Memorial Hospital
Associate Professor of Orthopaedic Surgery
Northwestern University Medical School
Chicago, Illinois

"This book, *Torticollis: Differential Diagnosis, Assessment and Treatment, Surgical Management and Bracing,* is a compendium of concepts regarding torticollis of which all clinical practitioners should be aware. It brings together the multidisciplinary concept needed to assess and diagnose as well as to treat the infant and the older child with torticollis.

There still remain many unanswered questions regarding CMT but this book by Karen Karmel-Ross provides up-to-date explanations and treatment protocols which will be useful for the practicing physical and occupational therapist as well as orthopaedist."

Richard D. Beauchamp, MD, FRCSC
Clinical Professor, Department of Orthopaedic Surgery
University of British Columbia
Active Staff, Department of Paediatric Orthopaedic Surgery, British Columbia's Children's Hospital
Medical Director, Shriners Gait Lab
Sunny Hill Health Center for Children
Vancouver, British Columbia, Canada

"With timely expert medical care, most cases of congenital muscular torticollis can be resolved or dramatically improved. However, the best treatment approach involves a multidisciplinary team that provides swift referral, accurate orthopaedic assessment and differential diagnosis, specialized physical therapy treatment, and in some cases surgical interventions. Unfortunately, medical literature is rarely multidisciplinary, and it is surprisingly difficult to uncover invaluable reviews such as this on specific medical conditions. This text provides a comprehensive, state of the art review of this common musculoskeletal condition that would be extremely useful to family practice physicians and pediatricians, general and pediatric orthopaedists, or physical medicine and rehabilitation physicians who evaluate infants as part of their practice. It is especially helpful for physical therapists who previously would have to consult multiple sources when treating this disorder, and still be unsuccessful in finding the breadth of assessment and treatment information as incorporated in this volume. I believe that families, as consumers of health care and as shared decision makers in the medical management of their child, would also find this book exceptionally helpful and informative, and it would answer many of their questions and alleviate many of their concerns, while offering them an essential and active guide to treatment. The depth of description included here on the primary and secondary musculoskeletal deformities in CMT is unlikely to be found elsewhere in the medical literature. As a physical therapist who is also a faculty member in a Department of Orthopaedics, I would enthusiastically recommend this text to my surgical and non-surgical colleagues alike."

Diane L. Damiano, PhD, PT
Assistant Professor of Orthopaedics and Rehabilitation
Milton S. Hershey Medical Center
The Pennsylvania State University

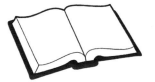

"**C**omprehensive management of the child with torticollis is multifaceted, requiring a team approach that utilizes the distinct expertise of physical therapists, pediatric surgeons (and in some cases, pediatric neurologists and ophthalmologists), and orthotists. This text, edited by a physical therapist with a great deal of clinical experience in the management of children with congenital muscular torticollis (CMT), clearly reflects the philosophy of the team approach by including contributions from a pediatric orthopedist, pediatric general surgeons, and several pediatric physical therapists.

The audience targeted by this text comes from several medical disciplines, and individuals involved in the care of children with torticollis will appreciate the articles contributed from outside of their own profession. Therapists will profit from the chapters generated by physicians reviewing the differential diagnosis and surgical management of CMT. Physicians will appreciate the chapters contributed by the physical therapists, which provide a detailed, comprehensive approach to the non-operative management of CMT. The chapter on the use of splinting describes three innovative designs that can be used in non-operative and post-operative settings. The chapter considering the relation between asymmetric head/neck positioning and postural development is particularly intriguing, underscoring the point that this deformity is not just cosmetic but may be associated with significant developmental deficits. The chapter on surgical management, which considers one type of distal unipolar release, is well written.

The multi-disciplinary nature of this text is its greatest strength. By bringing together a wide range of related materials under one cover, this text earns a place in the personal (or institutional) library of all individuals (or institutions) that care for children with torticollis."

Jon R. Davids, MD
Director
Motion Analysis Laboratory
Shriners Hospitals for Children
Greenville, South Carolina

"**T**his book covers a common, poorly understood and frequently misdiagnosed lesion, in a through and conise manner. The majority of infants with torticollis recover without the need for surgical intervention but the authors have given definitive indications when such therapy is required. The chapters dealing with torticollis recognition, active and passive exercises, and the use of bracing devices are well illustrated. Ms. Karmel-Ross's assessment, that more chronic follow-up for the long term effect of this lesion is needed, is very insightful since it comes from her unique experience with a very large population of these children. This is a potentially valuable source of information for all primary care pediatric physicians, nurse practitioners and physical therapists."

David L. Dudgeon, MD
Division Chief Pediatric Surgery
Rainbow Babies'
and Children's Hospital
University Hospitals of Cleveland

The Haworth Press, Inc.

Torticollis:
Differential Diagnosis,
Assessment and Treatment,
Surgical Management
and Bracing

Torticollis:
Differential Diagnosis, Assessment and Treatment, Surgical Management and Bracing

Karen Karmel-Ross
Editor

The Haworth Press, Inc.
New York • London

Torticollis: Differential Diagnosis, Assessment and Treatment, Surgical Management and Bracing has also been published as *Physical & Occupational Therapy in Pediatrics,* Volume 17, Number 2 1997.

Cover design by Thomas J. Mayshock Jr.

Cover Legend: Front, back, rotation left and rotation right view of a 9-month-old male with congenital muscular torticollis. Observe the plagiocephaly, developing hemihypoplasia, the decreased ability to rotate the head toward the involved side, and the left lateral neck flexion posture maintained during rotation of the head toward the noninvolved side.

The Haworth Press, Inc., 10 Alice Street, Binghamton, NY 13904-1580 USA

Library of Congress Cataloging-in-Publication Data

Torticollis : differential diagnosis, assessment and treatment, surgical management and bracing / Karen Karmel-Ross, editor.
     p. cm. – (Physical & occupational therapy in pediatrics ; v. 17, no. 2)
     Includes bibliographical references and index.
     ISBN 0-7890-0316-3 (alk. paper). – ISBN 0-7890-0317-1 (pbk.)
     1. Torticollis. 2. Children–Diseases. I. Karmel-Ross, Karen. II. Series.
     [DNLM: 1. Torticollis–diagnosis. 2. Torticollis–therapy. 3. Torticollis–surgery. 4. Diagnosis, Differential. W1 PH683M v. 17 no. 2 1997 / WE 708 T711 1997]
RJ482.T6T67 1997
618.92'7–dc21
DNLM/DLC
for Library of Congress
                                            97-10982
                                              CIP

This book is dedicated to the families and their children who will or have endured treatment for torticollis and to my family (Fred, Alexandra and Jacob) for their support.

Karen Karmel-Ross, PT, PCS, LMT

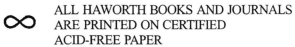

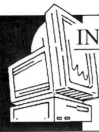

INDEXING & ABSTRACTING

Contributions to this publication are selectively indexed or abstracted in print, electronic, online, or CD-ROM version(s) of the reference tools and information services listed below. This list is current as of the copyright date of this publication. See the end of this section for additional notes.

- *Academic Abstracts/CD-ROM,* EBSCO Publishing Editorial Department, P.O. Box 590, Ipswich, MA 01938-0590

- *Biosciences Information Service of Biological Abstracts (BIOSIS),* Biosciences Information Service, 2100 Arch Street, Philadelphia, PA 19103-1399

- *Child Development Abstracts & Bibliography,* University of Kansas, 2 Bailey Hall, Lawrence, KS 66045

- *CINAHL (Cumulative Index to Nursing & Allied Health Literature), in print, also on CD-ROM from CD PLUS, EBSCO, and SilverPlatter, and online from CDP Online (formerly BRS), Data-Star, and PaperChase. (Support materials include Subject Heading List, Database Search Guide, and instructional video),* CINAHL Information Systems, P.O. Box 871/1509 Wilson Terrace, Glendale, CA 91209-0871

- *CNPIEC Reference Guide: Chinese National Directory of Foreign Periodicals,* P.O. Box 88, Beijing, People's Republic of China

- *Developmental Medicine & Child Neurology,* Mac Keith Press, 526-529 High Holborn House, 52-54 High Holborn, London WC1V 6RL, England

- *Educational Administration Abstracts (EAA),* Sage Publications, Inc., 2455 Teller Road, Newbury Park, CA 91320

- *Exceptional Child Education Resources (ECER), (CD/ROM from SilverPlatter and hard copy),* The Council for Exceptional Children, 1920 Association Drive, Reston, VA 20191

(continued)

- *Excerpta Medica/Secondary Publishing Division,* Elsevier Science Inc., Secondary Publishing Division, 655 Avenue of the Americas, New York, NY 10010

- *Family Studies Database (online and CD/ROM),* National Information Services Corporation, 306 East Baltimore Pike, 2nd Floor, Media, PA 19063

- *Health Source: Indexing & Abstracting of 160 selected health related journals, updated monthly:* EBSCO Publishing, 83 Pine Street, Peabody, MA 01960

- *Health Source Plus: expanded version of "Health Source" to be released shortly:* EBSCO Publishing, 83 Pine Street, Peabody, MA 01960

- *INTERNET ACCESS (& additional networks) Bulletin Board for Libraries ("BUBL"), coverage of information resources on INTERNET, JANET, and other networks.*
  - JANET X.29: UK.AC.BATH.BUBL or 00006012101300
  - TELNET: BUBL.BATH.AC.UK or 138.38.32.45 login 'bubl'
  - Gopher: BUBL.BATH.AC.UK (138.32.32.45). Port 7070
  - World Wide Web: http://www.bubl.bath.ac.uk./BUBL/home.html
  - NISSWAIS: telnetniss.ac.uk (for the NISS gateway)
  The Andersonian Library, Curran Building, 101 St. James Road, Glasgow G4 ONS, Scotland

- *Occupational Therapy Database (OTDBASE),* 3485 Point Grey Road, Vancouver, BC V6R 1A6, Canada

- *Occupational Therapy Index,* British Library Medical Information Service, Boston Spa, Wetherby, West Yorkshire, LS23 7BQ, United Kingdom

- *OT BibSys,* American Occupational Therapy Foundation, P.O. Box 31220, Rockville, MD 20824-1220

- *Sage Family Studies Abstracts (SFSA),* Sage Publications, Inc., 2455 Teller Road, Newbury Park, CA 91320

- *Sage Urban Studies Abstracts (SUSA),* Sage Publications, Inc., 2455 Teller Road, Newbury Park, CA 91320

(continued)

- ***Social Work Abstracts,*** National Association of Social Workers, 750 First Street NW, 8th Floor, Washington, DC 20002

- ***Sport Database/Discus,*** Sport Information Resource Center, 1600 James Naismith Drive, Suite 107, Gloucester, Ontario K1B 5N4, Canada

- ***Violence and Abuse Abstracts: A Review of Current Literature on Interpersonal Violence (VAA),*** Sage Publications, Inc., 2455 Teller Road, Newbury Park, CA 91320

SPECIAL BIBLIOGRAPHIC NOTES

*related to special journal issues (separates)
and indexing/abstracting*

❑ indexing/abstracting services in this list will also cover material in any "separate" that is co-published simultaneously with Haworth's special thematic journal issue or DocuSerial. Indexing/abstracting usually covers material at the article/chapter level.

❑ monographic co-editions are intended for either non-subscribers or libraries which intend to purchase a second copy for their circulating collections.

❑ monographic co-editions are reported to all jobbers/wholesalers/approval plans. The source journal is listed as the "series" to assist the prevention of duplicate purchasing in the same manner utilized for books-in-series.

❑ to facilitate user/access services all indexing/abstracting services are encouraged to utilize the co-indexing entry note indicated at the bottom of the first page of each article/chapter/contribution.

❑ this is intended to assist a library user of any reference tool (whether print, electronic, online, or CD-ROM) to locate the monographic version if the library has purchased this version but not a subscription to the source journal.

❑ individual articles/chapters in any Haworth publication are also available through the Haworth Document Delivery Services (HDDS).

Torticollis:
Differential Diagnosis,
Assessment and Treatment,
Surgical Management and Bracing

CONTENTS

ABOUT THE EDITOR

Karen Karmel-Ross, PT, PCS, LMT, is Clinical Specialist in the Department of Rehabilitation Services at Rainbow Babies' and Children's Hospital of the University Hospitals of Cleveland in Ohio. Board-certified in pediatric physical therapy with the American Board of Physical Therapy Specialties, she has published research regarding the effects of Neuromuscular Electrical Stimulation (NMES) on the strength and function of children with spina bifida and has lectured nationally on congenital muscular torticollis. She recently developed a longitudinal database for University Hospitals of Cleveland's Pediatric Neuromuscular Clinic and is currently developing a range-of-motion measurement device for children with torticollis. Ms. Karmel-Ross is a graduate of the eight-week Pediatric Neurodevelopmental Treatment (NDT) course and has an Ohio medical license for massage therapy.

Preface

Torticollis describes an abnormal neck posture in which a lateral translation of the head on the trunk occurs in addition to variable degrees of lateral head tilt and neck rotation. As a result, the chin points to one side and up, with or without contracture of neck muscles on the contralateral side. Torticollis is not a diagnosis but rather a sign of an underlying disorder. A search of the literature revealed over 1,500 articles that discuss or make reference to torticollis. A review of this literature reveals no agreement as to etiology, treatment, or even terminology. Muscular torticollis is the third most common congenital musculoskeletal anomaly after dislocated hip and clubfoot, with reports of incidence varying from 0.04% to 1.9%.[1,2]

The purpose of this volume is to share information on clinical management of infants and children with torticollis by physicians, surgeons, and therapists. The volume covers the following areas:

- Differential Diagnosis of Torticollis
- Literature Review of Conservative Management of Torticollis
- Assessment and Treatment Strategies for Infants and Children with Torticollis
- Interventions Including Surgery and Bracing
- The Effect of Asymmetrical Posture on Sensory Organization and Motor Skill Development

Treatment for torticollis is controversial. A search for a diagnosis when torticollis posture is encountered is critical in determining

---

[Haworth co-indexing entry note]: "Preface." Karmel-Ross, Karen. Co-published simultaneously in *Physical & Occupational Therapy in Pediatrics* (The Haworth Press, Inc.) Vol. 17, No. 2, 1997, pp. xiii-xiv; and: *Torticollis: Differential Diagnosis, Assessment and Treatment, Surgical Management and Bracing* (ed: Karen Karmel-Ross) The Haworth Press, Inc., 1997, pp. xiii-xiv. Single or multiple copies of this article are available for a fee from The Haworth Document Delivery Service [1-800-342-9678, 9:00 a.m. - 5:00 p.m. (EST). E-mail address: getinfo@haworth.com].

appropriate treatment. It is important to recognize the impact of this disorder on the growth and development of the child and the urgency for early intervention when congenital muscular torticollis (CMT) is appreciated. Conservative treatment is reported to be effective in > 80% of the cases of CMT if treatment is initiated under one year of age.[3-6]

Nevertheless, many authors in the literature on torticollis have observed that musculoskeletal sequelae persist despite early treatment. Craniofacial asymmetry, intermittent head tilt, and scoliosis are the observations most often cited.[1,3-5]

I hope this volume will serve as a reminder that the etiology of CMT remains obscure, that the treatment of an infant or child with torticollis posture should not begin until a diagnosis for this disorder has been identified, that a comprehensive conservative approach to treatment initiated as early as possible can be functionally effective, and that successful management of persistent torticollis requires much more than changing the restrictions of movement in the cervical spine.

Karen Karmel-Ross

REFERENCES

1. Coventry MB, Harris LE. Congenital muscular torticollis in infancy: some observations regarding treatment. *J Bone Joint Surg.* 1959; 41:815-822.

2. Suzuki S, Yamamura T, Fujita A. An etiological relationship between congenital torticollis and obstetrical paralysis. *Int Orthop.* 1984; 8:175-181.

3. Binder H, Eng GD, Gaiser JF, Koch B. Congenital muscular torticollis results of conservative management with long-term follow-up in 85 cases. *Arch Phys Med Rehab.* 1987; 68:222-225.

4. Canal ST, Griffin DW, Hubbard CN. Congenital muscular torticollis. *J Bone Joint Surg.* 1982; 64:810-816.

5. MacDonald D. Sternomastoid tumor and muscular torticollis. *J Bone Joint Surg.* 1969; 51:432-443.

6. Emery C. The determinants of treatment duration for congenital muscular torticollis. *Phys Ther* 1994; 74:921-929.

The Differential Diagnosis of Torticollis in Children

Daniel R. Cooperman

SUMMARY. Torticollis is a term that describes asymmetrical posturing of the head and neck. The majority of children who present with torticollis during the first year of life have congenital muscular torticollis (CMT) secondary to unilateral fibrosis of the sternocleidomastoid muscle. Observation alone leads to residual deformity in up to 20% of these children, but aggressive treatment of CMT improves outcome. One in five children presenting with torticollis have a non-muscular etiology with either soft tissue involvement or bony involvement. Other diagnoses associated with torticollis include benign paroxysmal torticollis, congenital absence of one or more cervical muscles, Klippel-Feil syndrome, hemivertebrae, or other congenital anomalies of the cervical spine. Acquired torticollis may be secondary to trauma, or children can develop torticollis secondary to inflammatory conditions such as pharyngitis. Torticollis is also seen in response to certain ocular lesions as well as in children with symptomatic hiatal hernias. The most dangerous cause of non-muscular acquired torticollis is related to neurologic syndromes, such as syringomyelia, dystonic or post-encephalitic syndromes, herniated cervical discs, and, especially, posterior fossa pathology. In a large series of children with non-muscular torticollis, 10% resulted from neurologic problems, half of which involved tumors. When torticollis is encountered, a search for a diagnosis should begin. After a

---

Daniel R. Cooperman, MD, is Associate Professor of Orthopaedics, Case Western Reserve University, Cleveland, OH.

Address correspondence to: Daniel R. Cooperman, MD, 11100 Euclid Avenue, Cleveland, OH 44106.

[Haworth co-indexing entry note]: "The Differential Diagnosis of Torticollis in Children." Cooperman, Daniel R. Co-published simultaneously in *Physical & Occupational Therapy in Pediatrics* (The Haworth Press, Inc.) Vol. 17, No. 2, 1997, pp. 1-11; and: *Torticollis: Differential Diagnosis, Assessment and Treatment, Surgical Management and Bracing* (ed: Karen Karmel-Ross) The Haworth Press, Inc., 1997, pp. 1-11. Single or multiple copies of this article are available for a fee from The Haworth Document Delivery Service [1-800-342-9678, 9:00 a.m. - 5:00 p.m. (EST). E-mail address: getinfo@haworth.com].

1

diagnosis is made, treatment can begin. *[Article copies available for a fee from The Haworth Document Delivery Service: 1-800-342-9678. E-mail address: getinfo@haworth.com]*

The term torticollis is derived from two Latin terms, *tortus,* meaning twisted, and *collum,* meaning neck. Any asymmetrical posturing of the head and neck is torticollis. Unfortunately the term has become synonymous with congenital muscular torticollis (CMT). This sometimes leads to confusion when the word is used. Although CMT is the most common cause of torticollis, it is not the only cause. This article discusses CMT and other causes of torticollis and provides information on differential diagnosis.

CONGENITAL TORTICOLLIS

Etiology, Pathology and Imaging in CMT

Congenital Muscular Torticollis is a condition caused by unilateral fibrosis of the sternocleidomastoid (SCM) muscle. The etiology of the SCM fibrosis is unknown. For centuries this condition has been seen in children who were the products of difficult labors and deliveries. As a result, it has been suggested that direct trauma to the SCM during delivery causes muscle damage and the subsequent fibrosis seen in CMT. Other authorities disagree. As examples of the controversy, Lidge and associates[1] and Jones[2] present a wide ranging historical review of the etiology of CMT discussing arguments that favor direct injury to the SCM, ischemic injury based on abnormal vascular patterns, rupture of the muscle and infective myositis. They also discuss neurogenic injury, hereditary factors and anlage defect. Recently Davids and colleagues[3] suggested that SCM fibrosis may be the result of an intrauterine compartment syndrome due to extreme head posturing within the birth canal. Little agreement exists on the etiology of SCM fibrosis in CMT, although there is agreement that SCM fibrosis causes CMT.

A majority of patients with CMT evidence a tumor in the SCM muscle during the first 3 months of life. Jones[2] followed 99 CMT patients for 6 years and reported that SCM tumors appeared in 2/3 of the patients. The average time of appearance was at 3.5 weeks of age (range: birth to 3 months). Published reports of biopsy in CMT are reasonably consistent.[4] Biopsies of the tumors reveal the histologic appearance of a fibroma. In children with CMT, both with and without the tumor, extensive fibrosis surrounds the muscle fibers (endomysial fibrosis). No evidence of hematoma or infection within the muscle, or arterial or venous abnormalities exists. On electromicrographic assessment, non-specific degeneration is noted. Davids and associates[3] suggest that histochemical studies reveal evidence of nerve degeneration and varying amounts of reinnervation.

Chan and associates[5] recently reported an ultrasound study of CMT in 36 children, 28 of whom had tumors on clinical exam while eight did not. He noted that all had tumors revealed by ultrasound, usually in the middle or lower third of the SCM muscle. The ultrasonic pattern was complex. Some images had homogeneous echogenic patterns while others had mixed hyper-, iso- and hypo-echoic patterns, with or without evidence of calcification.

Davids, Wenger and Mubarak[3] presented magnetic resonance imaging (MRI) results on nine infants with classical CMT, four with palpable masses in the SCM muscle and five without. All nine had an abnormal MRI signal throughout the entire affected muscle. None had discrete masses that could be isolated. The affected SCM muscle had a diameter that was two to four times greater than the opposite normal SCM muscle. The authors suggest that these changes are similar to those in MRI scans of the legs and forearms of patients with compartment syndromes.[6-8] They postulate that classical CMT is the result of a compartment syndrome within the SCM muscle compartment caused by extreme forward flexion, lateral bending, and rotation of the infant's head within the birth canal. Kinking of the mid-substance of the ipsilateral SCM muscle is postulated to lead to an ischemic injury. As in compartment syndromes in other locations, ischemic injury results in nerve and muscle damage, followed by massive swelling. Damaged muscle fibers would then be replaced by fibrous tissue accompanied by varying amounts of nerve degeneration and regeneration over time. The authors note that these findings are consistent with the pathologic data available. Their hypothesis is presently the most attractive etiologic explanation for CMT.

Clinical Features of CMT

CMT is a condition produced by unilateral fibrosis of the sterno-cleidomastoid muscle (SCM). The contracture which results causes an asymmetrical posture of the head and neck. The ear is tilted toward the side of the shortened muscle and the chin is rotated toward the opposite side. Neck rotation toward the affected side is limited. Over a few to six months in 10% to 20% of untreated patients marked deformity results, including fixed, restricted ipsilateral neck rotation, ipsilateral face and contralateral skull flattening (plagiocephaly), and hemihypoplasia.[1,2]

The incidence of CMT reported in the literature varies between 0.084%[9] and 1.9%.[10] Coventry and associates[11] suggest an incidence of 0.4% based on 35 cases found in 7,835 babies at the Mayo Clinic who were born in the local region. All of these infants had tumors in the SCM muscle. The male to female ratio was almost equal.

Infants with CMT frequently have associated problems, including hip dysplasia, club foot, metatarsus adductus, and brachial plexus injury. In 1982 Morrison and MacEwan[12] reported on 232 patients with CMT; 32 had hip dysplasia with ten unilateral and five bilateral dislocations. In addition, four infants had unilateral and seven bilateral metatarsus adductus, and one had a unilateral clubfoot. Binder and colleagues[13] suggested that the incidence of hip dysplasia increases with the severity of the torticollis. Five of 21 patients with severe torticollis in her sample of 277 patients had hip dysplasia.

Differential Diagnosis of Congenital Torticollis

The diagnosis of CMT is usually made upon physical examination during the first few months of life. Babies present with a tumor or a tight band in the SCM muscle. The child may develop a head tilt and limited neck rotation. Many children, however, present with torticollis without a tumor, and a thorough evaluation must be undertaken to determine the cause of the torticollis posture.

Recently Ballock and Song[14] reviewed 288 patients with torticollis referred to the Texas Scottish-Rite Hospital for Children. One in five (53/288) had a non-muscular etiology. Klippel-Feil syndrome or congenital scoliosis or both were seen in 16 patients (5.8% of the entire presenting group of 288 patients). An underlying neurologic disorder was present in 27 children (9.4%), including ocular disorder in 12, brachial plexus damage in 9, and central nervous system (CNS) lesions in 6 patients. The latter included one astrocytoma of the brainstem and spinal cord, a ganglioglioma of the cerebellum, a glioma of the brainstem, an arachnoid cyst in the parietal lobe, agenesis of the cerebellar hemisphere, and congenital cystic brain anomalies. Finally, torticollis was also noted in two patients each with inflammatory illnesses, atlanto-axial rotary subluxation, and clavicle fractures.

Ballock's and Song's data[14] underscore the importance of establishing an etiology for torticollis before beginning treatment because torticollis is not synonymous with SCM muscle contracture. Many lesions can masquerade as classical congenital muscular torticollis, so a good examination is necessary to establish the etiology of torticollis before treatment is begun. The initial examination should include a history and a physical examination. The history will determine if the lesion is congenital or acquired and, if acquired, whether traumatic or non-traumatic in origin. The physical examination will determine whether there is an SCM muscle contracture, whether neck range of motion is limited, and if other health problems are present. If neck motion is restricted, an x-ray will determine if congenital anomalies of the spine are causing the torticollis. No treatment for restricted range of neck rotation should begin until an x-ray of the cervical spine is taken and an active search for the etiology of torticollis is complete.

We divide congenital torticollis into four general categories:

1. Torticollis with unilateral SCM muscle contracture and a tumor during the first 3 months of life with an otherwise normal x-ray. This is the most classic presentation of CMT.
2. Torticollis with SCM muscle contracture without a tumor in the SCM and with a normal x-ray. This can be classic CMT where the tumor is not observed or classic CMT in which no palpable tumor forms.
3. Head and neck asymmetry similar in appearance to classic CMT without SCM contracture and with normal x-rays. Causes include:

   a. Benign paroxysmal torticollis beginning in the first few months of life. The torticollis can alternate between right-sided and left-sided, is worse in the morning than at night, and resolves spontaneously at about a year of age.[15,16]

b. Congenital absence of one or several cervical muscles or of the transverse ligament.[17]
c. Contracture of other neck muscles including scalenus anterior, omohyoid, or trapezius.
d. Generalized neck contractures as a result of abnormal, delayed neuromuscular development.

4. Congenital torticollis with abnormal spinal x-rays. Klippel-Feil syndrome (Figure 1, all Figures cited are in the Appendix) and congenital scoliosis (Figure 2) were noted in 5.8% of the patients reviewed by Ballock and Song.[14] Among the causes of congenital scoliosis are hemivertebrae, unilateral atlanto-occipital fusions, and bar formation. Unilateral absence of a C-1 facet and basilar impression can also result in torticollis.

ACQUIRED TORTICOLLIS

Acquired torticollis has a multiplicity of possible causes. Torticollis may result from almost any disturbance of the muscles or bones of the skull and cervical spine, any abnormalities in the brain or spinal cord areas related to head and neck posture, or any ocular disturbance producing diplopia. In addition, psychiatric and pharmacologic causes of torticollis exist. The following list describes some of the frequently encountered causes of acquired torticollis.

1. Acquired torticollis following a history of trauma with or without bony lesions. Acute trauma resulting in fracture to the head, neck, clavicle or scapula can result in torticollis due to muscle spasm. Neck trauma may result in fracture of the dens or lateral masses of the atlas, rotary subluxation of C-1 on C-2 (Figure 3), or unilateral subluxation of C-2 on C-3.[18] Soft tissue injuries of the SCM muscle resulting in hematoma within the muscle or acute rupture of the muscle can also cause torticollis.[19]
2. Acquired torticollis, non-traumatic, resulting in bony deformity. Rotary subluxation of C-1 on C-2 is often seen in inflammatory conditions. These include osteomyelitis of the cervical spine, rheumatoid arthritis, and cervical lymphadenitis, as well as pharyngitis, tonsillitis, mastoiditis, and cervical ab-

scess. Usually the subluxation resolves as inflammation subsides. Occasionally, the subluxation becomes fixed, necessitating active treatment including bracing, traction and even spinal fusion.[20-22]

3. Acquired torticollis, non-traumatic without fixed bony deformity. Often a specialty consult (Pediatric Surgery, Ophthalmology or Neurology) is needed to arrive at the following diagnoses:

   a. Ocular lesions can cause torticollis,[23] including melanoblastoma of the choroid, eye muscle paralysis, thrombosis of the inferior temporal retinal vein, and acute defects secondary to retinal detachment. Congenital nystagmus and diplopia also can cause torticollis.
   b. Sandifer Syndrome is a rare cause of torticollis related to hiatal hernia. Approximately one case of Sandifer syndrome occurs for every 100 children with symptomatic hiatal hernia.[24]
   c. Neurological syndromes[22,25] resulting in torticollis include:

      1. Arnold-Chiari malformation and syringomyelia, especially related to scoliosis
      2. Dystonic syndromes
      3. Postencephalitis syndromes
      4. Herniated cervical disk
      5. Posterior fossa pathology

   The diagnosis is suspected on neurologic exam and confirmed on MRI. Ballock and Song[14] noted 6 CNS defects in 288 children referred for torticollis.

4. Acquired painful torticollis may result from:
   a. Osteoid osteoma
   b. Osteoblastoma

   Bone scan may be helpful in diagnosis.

In summary, torticollis is a term describing a twisted head and neck. It is not synonymous with CMT. When torticollis is encountered, a search for a diagnosis should begin. After a diagnosis is made, appropriate treatment can begin.

REFERENCES

1. Lidge RT, Bechtol RC, Lambert CN. Congenital muscular torticollis. Etiology and pathology. *J Bone Joint Surg.* 1957; 39-A:1165-1181.

2. Jones PG. *Torticollis in Infancy and Childhood.* Springfield, IL: Charles C Thomas, Publisher; 1968.

3. Davids JR, Wenger DR, Mubarak SJ. Congenital muscular torticollis: sequela of intrauterine or perinatal compartment syndrome. *J Pediatr Ortho.* 1993; 13:141-147.

4. Tachdjian M. *Pediatric Orthopaedics.* Philadelphia, PA: WB Saunders Company; 1972.

5. Chan YL, Cheng JCY, Metreweli C. Ultrasonography of congenital muscular torticollis. *Pediatr Radiology.* 1992; 22:356-360.

6. DeSmet AA, Fisher DR, Heiner JP, Keene JS. Magnetic resonance imaging of muscle tears. *Skel Radiol.* 1990; 19:283-286.

7. Deutsch AL, Mink JH. Magnetic resonance imaging of musculoskeletal injuries. *Radiol Clin North Am.* 1989; 27:983-1002.

8. Fleckenstein JL, Weatherall PT, Parkey RW, Payne JA, Peshock RM. Sports related muscle injuries: evaluation with MR imaging. *Radiology.* 1989; 72:793-798.

9. Ling CM, Low YS: Sternomastoid tumor and muscular torticollis. *Clin Orthop.* 1972; 86:144-150.

10. Suzuki S, Yamamura T, Fujita A. Aetiological relationship between congenital torticollis and obstetrical paralysis. *Int Orthop.* 1984; 8:175-181.

11. Coventry MB, Harris LE, Bianco AJ, Bulbulian AH. Congenital muscular torticollis (wryneck). *Postgrad Med.* 1960; 28:383-392.

12. Morrison DL, MacEwen GD. Congenital muscular torticollis: observations regarding clinical findings, associated conditions and results of treatment. *J Pediatr Ortho.* 1982;2:500-505.

13. Binder H, Eng GD, Gaiser JF, Koch B. Congenital muscular torticollis, results of conservative management with long-term follow-up in 85 cases. *Arch Phys Med Rehabil.* 1987; 68:222-225.

14. Ballock RT, Song KM. The prevalence of non-muscular causes of torticollis in children. Personal Communication.

15. Bolton PS. Torticollis: a review of etiology, pathology, diagnosis and treatment. *J Manipul Physiolog Therapeutics.* 1985; 8:29-32.

16. Bratt HD, Menelaus MB. Benign paroxysmal torticollis of infancy. *J Bone Joint Surg.* 1992; 74-B:449-451.

17. Clark RN. Diagnosis and management of torticollis. *Pediatr Annals.* 1976; 5:43-57.

18. Hahn ML, Davidson R, Drummond DS. Acquired torticollis in children. *Ortho Review.* 1991; XX:667-674.

19. Schuyler-Hacker H, Green R, Wingate L, Sklar J. Acute torticollis secondary to rupture of the sternocleidomastoid. *Arch Phys Med Rehabil.* 1989; 70:851-853.

20. Tom LWC, Rossiter JL, Sutton LN, Davidson RS, Potsic WP. Torticollis in children. *Otolaryn Head Neck Surg.* 1991; 105:1-5.

21. Bredenkamp JK, Maceri DR. Inflammatory torticollis in children. *Arch Otolar Head Neck Surg.* 1990; 116:310-313.

22. Kiwak KJ. Establishing an etiology for torticollis. *Postgrad Med.* 1984; 75:126-134.

23. Spielmann A. Congenital nystagmus: clinical types and their surgical treatment. *Ophthalmolog Basel.* 1981; 182:65-72.

24. O'Donnell JJ, Howard RO. Torticollis associated with hiatus hernia. *Amer J Ophthal.* 1971; 71:1134-1137.

25. Turgut M, Akalan N, Bertan V, Erbengi A, Eryilmaz M. Acquired torticollis as the only presenting symptom in children with posterior fossa tumors. *Child's Nerv Syst.* 1995; 11:86-88.

APPENDIX

FIGURE 1. Klippel-Feil syndrome is a rare congenital anomaly in which one or more vertebrae in the cervical region are fused. Inappropriate fusion of C-2, C-3 and C-4 is shown in this x-ray.

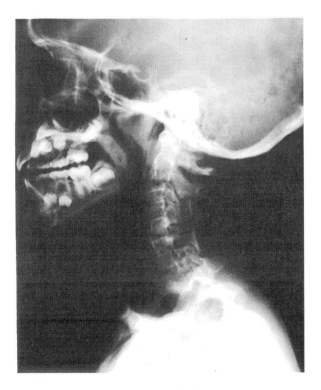

APPENDIX (continued)

FIGURE 2. Hemivertebrae formation is one cause of cervical scoliosis which can lead to torticollis. Note the hemivertebrae between C-2 and C-3 as well as the hemivertebrae at the base of the cervical spine causing this cervical scoliosis.

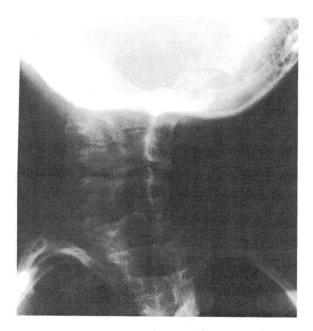

FIGURE 3. Rotary subluxation of C-1 on C-2 is an uncommon upper cervical subluxation. In this tomogram the base of the skull and the dens of C-2 are clearly seen. The two lateral masses are asymmetrically placed with respect to the dens with the left hand lateral mass much closer to the dens than the right hand lateral mass. This asymmetrical relationship can be well appreciated using either a linear tomography or a computed tomography scan.

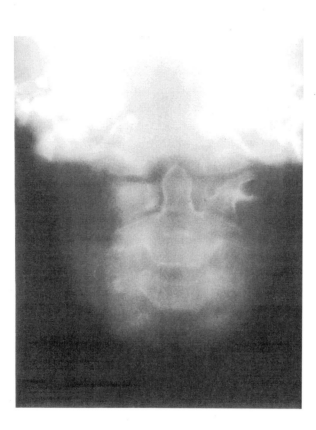

Conservative Management
of Congenital Muscular Torticollis:
A Literature Review

Carolyn Emery

SUMMARY. This article provides a review of the literature on the conservative management of congenital muscular torticollis. Variations among studies are found in physiotherapeutic regime, definition of outcomes, and results. All authors, however, report good (mild facial asymmetry, tilt or range restriction) to excellent (full neck range of motion, no facial asymmetry) outcomes for the vast majority of patients who receive conservative management of congenital muscular torticollis. Overall, fewer than about 16% of those treated before one year of age require surgical intervention. *[Article copies available for a fee from The Haworth Document Delivery Service: 1-800-342-9678. E-mail address: getinfo@haworth.com]*

Congenital muscular torticollis (CMT) is an asymmetrical posture of the head and neck caused by unilateral fibrosis of the sternocleidomastoid (SCM) muscle (see Cooperman, this volume, for information on differential diagnosis). Numerous reports on the outcomes of conservative management of CMT have appeared in

Carolyn Emery, BScPT, is Physiotherapy Consultant, Max Bell Sports Medicine Physiotherapy Centre, Calgary, Alberta, Canada.

Address correspondence to: Carolyn Emery, Max Bell Sports Medicine Physiotherapy Centre, 1001 Barlow Trail SE, Calgary, Alberta, Canada T2E 6S2.

[Haworth co-indexing entry note]: "Conservative Management of Congenital Muscular Torticollis: A Literature Review." Emery, Carolyn. Co-published simultaneously in *Physical & Occupational Therapy in Pediatrics* (The Haworth Press, Inc.) Vol. 17, No. 2, 1997, pp. 13-20; and: *Torticollis: Differential Diagnosis, Assessment and Treatment, Surgical Management and Bracing* (ed: Karen Karmel-Ross) The Haworth Press, Inc., 1997, pp. 13-20. Single or multiple copies of this article are available for a fee from The Haworth Document Delivery Service [1-800-342-9678, 9:00 a.m. - 5:00 p.m. (EST). E-mail address: getinfo@haworth.com].

the clinical literature,[1-6] and a number of specific physiotherapeutic treatment regimes are outlined by the authors of these clinical studies. The generally accepted components of conservative treatment include passive SCM muscle stretching exercises (i.e., ipsilateral rotation and contralateral lateral flexion), active range of motion (ROM) activities, positioning and handling techniques for postural correction, and lateral head righting strengthening exercises. Only the studies that systematically document outcomes of these conservative treatment regimes will be more closely reviewed in this article.

REVIEW OF THE LITERATURE

Although the treatments differ and none of these studies includes true control groups to rule out the effects of maturation and natural recovery, the results of conservative treatment suggest that surgery is seldom needed when patients are identified and treated early. Unfortunately, patients were identified at a variety of ages and the definitions of treatment outcomes also differ, making it difficult to compare the results of the various studies. In general, however, the definition of an "excellent" outcome typically includes no facial asymmetry and full neck ROM. "Good" outcome may include mild head tilt, asymmetry, or limited range, although "mild" is not specifically defined. "Satisfactory" or "fair" outcome includes both mild facial asymmetry and SCM hypoextensibility. "Poor" outcome is generally agreed to include persistent contracture of the SCM muscle with facial asymmetry. When surgery is listed as an outcome of unsuccessful conservative treatment, it is frequently listed as having been done "as required" without providing specific criteria. In Table 1, which summarizes the outcomes reported in the clinical literature, the specific definitions used by each author in reporting results are given.

To summarize, all of the studies reviewed report good to excellent results with conservative management of CMT. It should be noted, however, that Emery's study was the only prospective study among those reviewed.[4] None of the studies included controls for the possible effects of natural recovery or maturation on outcome, and none assigned subjects to treatment regimes systematically so

TABLE 1. Review of Literature on Conservative Management of Congenital Muscular Torticollis

Author/Yr. Study Type	Population	Treatment	Outcome*	Conclusions
Ling and Low[5] 1972 Retrospective comparison between infants with or without fibrotic mass in SCM	150 Ss: Group A (78%)- with fibrotic mass (70% <2 mos. at initial dx) Group B (22%)- no mass (43% <1 yr. at initial dx)	Frequent stretching by parents (technique not well defined) Surgery "if required" (mean age 7 yrs.)	Group A- Mean tx duration = 7 mos. 77% satisfactory 23% poor 98% stretching only, 2% surgery Group B- 50% satisfactory, 50% poor 50% stretching only, 42% surgery, 8% declined surgery	Conservative management in most cases of SCM mass is adequate. In patients > 6 mos. with no mass, surgery is tx of choice as success with stretches was poor and facial asymmetry was poorly corrected with delayed surgery.

* Satisfactory = normal or mild facial asymmetry with mild tightness of SCM. Poor = severe facial asymmetry with progression to muscular torticollis (i.e., hypoextensibility of SCM with no mass).

Author/Yr. Study Type	Population	Treatment	Outcome**	Conclusions
Morrison and MacEwen[6] 1982 Descriptive report on infants with varying age at dx	232 Ss: Time of Dx 43% at birth 21% <3 wks. 18% 3 wks.-3 mos. 15% >3 mos.	Stretches by parents at diaper change (combined movements: rotation/ lateral flexion in neutral, flexion & extension) Heat/massage Positioning Surgery "if required" (mean age 7.5 yrs.)	16% required surgery (36% excellent, 59% good, 5% poor results) 84% treated conservatively (71% excellent, 29% good, 0% poor results)	Good to excellent results with conservative rx if dx prior to 1 yr

** Excellent = no mass, no apparent deformity of neck, no head tilt, no asymmetry of face or skull, and full ROM. Good = same as excellent result but mild persistence of head tilt and/or facial asymmetry. Poor = persistent contracture of SCM, head tilt, facial and/or skull asymmetry with restriction of ROM.

TABLE 1 (continued)

Author/Yr. Study Type	Population	Treatment	Outcome	Conclusions
Binder et al.[1] 1987 Descriptive report of outcomes	277 Ss: 38.6% fibrotic mass, 81.6% <6 months at initial visit	Stretching by parents (SCM, upper trapezius, ipsilateral trunk muscles) Positioning/ handling to encourage active rotation Soft collar if head tilt >45 degrees Surgery "if required in moderate to severe cases"	70% resolution*** prior to 1 yr. regardless of severity or presence of fibrotic mass 5% surgical intervention	Authors interpreted their results to indicate that severity of restricted ROM and age at which treatment was initiated were key predictors of outcome. Resolution greater in mild to moderate cases when fibrotic mass present.

*** Resolution = Full passive lateral flexion and rotation easily achieved; child's head position in midline with the chin pointing forward.

Author/Yr. Study Type	Population	Treatment	Outcome	Conclusions
Cameron et al.[2] 1989 Comparison of groups < and > 3 mos. of age at initiation of rx	126 Ss <u>Group A</u> <3 mos. at rx initiation <u>Group B</u> >3 mos. at rx initiation	Stretching by parents 10X twice daily, rotation only. Surgery for a contracture which did not improve with passive stretching exercise	<u>Group A</u> 65% excellent,**** 27% good, 8% fair 0% surgery <u>Group B</u> 45% surgery	Success of passive stretching exercises is related to age at initiation of rx

**** Excellent = full rotation with no facial asymmetry. Good = full rotation with mild facial asymmetry or mild limitation of rotation with no facial asymmetry. Fair = mild limitation in rotation with mild facial asymmetry.

Author/Yr. Study Type	Population	Treatment	Outcome*****	Conclusions
de Chalain and Katz[3] 1992 Descriptive report comparing outcomes of rx initiated before 3 mos. and before 9 mos.	134 Ss: 67% < 3 mos. at rx initiation 100% < 9 mos. at rx initiation	Stretching exercises taught to mother: both rotation and side flexion, frequency not defined Surgery required "if not sufficient outcome"	60% improved sufficiently to warrant discharge, 36% defaulted from clinic, 4% surgery (mean age 2.4 yrs.)	Good results achieved with physical therapy begun before 3 mos. Indication for surgery: failure to improve with 3-6 mos. of rx or the appearance of facial asymmetry

***** Sufficient outcome = significant improvement in neck mobility within 3-6 mo. of physical therapy trial (providing that facial asymmetry is not yet present).

Author/Yr. Study Type	Population	Treatment	Outcome******	Conclusions
Emery[4] 1994 Prospective study of cohort entering rx with specific inclusion criteria	101 Ss: mean age = 4 mos. at rx initiation (25% fibrotic mass, 75% no mass)	Stretching by parents twice daily: rotation and lateral flexion 5X, 10 sec. holds Positioning/handling to encourage active rotation Tubular orthosis (TOT) if head tilt > 6 degrees (30% of Ss)	1 surgery, > 99% full recovery (Mean rx duration): 4.7 mos. (mass = 6.9 mos., no mass = 3.9 mos.); TOT group = 7.2 mos., no TOT = 3.6 mos.	Severity of restriction in rotation is key predictor of rx duration in no mass group. Both increased severity and presence of a fibrotic mass led to longer treatment duration. Age at initiation of treatment is unrelated to treatment duration if < 1 year.

****** Full recovery denotes full passive neck ROM in lateral flexion and rotation, and no residual head tilt. An equation to determine treatment duration in children with no mass present at initial assessment was statistically derived: $y = -.012x + .824$, where x = treatment duration (months) and y = severity of restriction in rotation (rotation to affected side/rotation to unaffected side).

that intervention variables could be compared. Furthermore, there do not appear to be consistently agreed-upon definitions of various degrees of successful outcome, and consistent criteria for identifying the need for surgical intervention are unavailable. Despite the shortcomings of reports of clinical interventions that lack experimental controls for alternative explanations of results, all of the authors suggest that early initiation of treatment is essential to successful outcome.

In addition to lack of experimental controls for threats to validity of study design, the differences among studies in success rates of conservative treatment may be partially explained by the characteristics of the samples of children examined and the inclusion criteria used in each study. Emery prospectively examined results in a clinical population of children who were referred to physical therapy for treatment with specific inclusion/exclusion criteria. Emery's[4] criteria for enrolling children in treatment were:

1. Diagnosed with CMT and referred by family physician, pediatrician or orthopaedic surgeon.
2. Initial assessment and initiation of treatment prior to 2 years of age.
3. Restricted neck ROM in lateral flexion or rotation or both.
4. Compliance with attending follow-up appointments once every two weeks (monthly after achievement of full passive neck ROM).

Excluded were children whose treatment was initiated at another facility, or who had medical complications that interfered with the standard treatment program, previous surgical correction of CMT, radiologic results indicating vertebral anomalies, ocular imbalance or nerve injury associated with CMT, or diagnosed or suspected syndromes, such as Down syndrome.

Emery demonstrated 99% resolution (i.e., full passive neck ROM in lateral flexion and rotation and no residual head tilt) without surgery.[4] The success rates of conservative management in the other studies reviewed were not as high, but the study samples included children with CMT examined at a surgical clinic with less stringent inclusion/exclusion criteria than Emery's.

The reports in the literature do not provide a clear answer to the question of whether the presence of a fibrotic SCM mass is a factor influencing the outcome of conservative treatment. Ling and Low reported better clinical results in the mass group with conservative treatment than in the no-mass group.[5] Binder and associates demonstrated 70% resolution of CMT prior to 1 year of age regardless of presence of fibrosis.[1] Finally, Emery demonstrated longer treatment durations in cases where there is presence of a mass.[4] Both Binder and associates[1] and Emery[4] scrutinized severity of restriction of ROM and agreed that severity is a key predictor of treatment duration.

Emery[4] presented a regression analysis to model severity of restriction in rotation and in lateral flexion, age at initiation of treatment, and presence of a fibrotic mass as a determinant of treatment duration. Only limitation in rotation (for the no-mass group) was a significant predictor. Children with a mass required longer treatment, regardless of severity of ROM restriction. Severity of restriction in rotation may be utilized to estimate treatment duration in children presenting with no mass using the equation described in Table 1. Severity of rotation was defined as the proportion of degrees toward the affected side divided by the degrees toward the unaffected side. For example, for a child with neck rotation limited to 75% of that on the contralateral side (severity = 0.75), the predicted treatment duration is 6.2 months.

CONCLUSION AND RECOMMENDATIONS

In summary, a review of the literature on CMT shows that fewer than about 16% of children treated conservatively before one year of age will require surgery. Typical treatment durations to produce complete neck mobility in this patient population ranged from 3-12 months.

Recommendations for future research include long-term followup studies to determine whether complete resolution of torticollis is maintained as the child grows. In addition, it is important to determine the rate of spontaneous recovery and identify criteria which may suggest that spontaneous recovery is likely. It would also be of interest to compare different frequencies or intensities of home treatment programming and their relative effects on speed or extent of recovery.

REFERENCES

1. Binder H, Eng G, Gaiser JF, Koch B. Congenital muscular torticollis: results of conservative management with long-term follow-up in 85 cases. *Arch Phys Med Rehabil.* 1987; 68:222-225.

2. Cameron BH, Cameron GS, Langer JC. Success of non-operative treatment for congenital muscular torticollis is dependent on early initiation of therapy. Presented at the Canadian Association of Paediatric Surgery, Quebec City, Quebec, Canada; September 1989.

3. de Chalain TMB, Katz A. Idiopathic muscular torticollis in children: the Cape Town experience. *Br J Plast Surg.* 1992; 45:297-301.

4. Emery C. The determinants of treatment duration for congenital muscular torticollis. *Phys Ther.* 1994; 74:921-929.

5. Ling CM, Low YS. Sternomastoid tumor and muscular torticollis. *Clin Orthop.* 1972; 86;144-150.

6. Morrison DL, MacEwen GD. Congenital muscular torticollis: observations regarding clinical findings, associated conditions and results of treatment. *J Pediatr Orthop.* 1982; 2:500-505.

Assessment and Treatment of Children with Congenital Muscular Torticollis

Karen Karmel-Ross
Michael Lepp

SUMMARY. The purpose of this article is to present a systematic approach to the assessment and treatment of children with congenital muscular torticollis. An assessment protocol and form, treatment pathways, and home program exercise sheets are provided in this article. *[Article copies available for a fee from The Haworth Document Delivery Service: 1-800-342-9678. E-mail address: getinfo@haworth.com]*

A distinct clinical entity seen in the newborn, infant, and child is muscular torticollis. Torticollis has been recognized for many centuries, but treatment and theories of its etiology remain controversial.

The usual clinical picture of congenital muscular torticollis (CMT) presents a newborn about two weeks of age with a tumor within the muscle belly of the sternocleidomastoid (SCM) muscle.

Karen Karmel-Ross, PT, PCS, LMT, is Pediatric Clinical Specialist, Department of Rehabilitation Services, University Hospitals of Cleveland, Cleveland, OH. Michael Lepp, PT, is in private practice, Associate Instructor of the Upledger Institute, and Clinical Instructor, Case Western Reserve University School of Dentistry, Cleveland, OH.

Address correspondence to: Karen Karmel-Ross, University Hospitals of Cleveland, Department of Rehabilitation Services, 11100 Euclid Avenue, Cleveland, OH 44106.

[Haworth co-indexing entry note]: "Assessment and Treatment of Children with Congenital Muscular Torticollis." Karmel-Ross, Karen, and Michael Lepp. Co-published simultaneously in *Physical & Occupational Therapy in Pediatrics* (The Haworth Press, Inc.) Vol. 17, No. 2, 1997, pp. 21-67; and: *Torticollis: Differential Diagnosis, Assessment and Treatment, Surgical Management and Bracing* (ed: Karen Karmel-Ross) The Haworth Press, Inc., 1997, pp. 21-67. Single or multiple copies of this article are available for a fee from The Haworth Document Delivery Service [1-800-342-9678, 9:00 a.m. - 5:00 p.m. (EST). E-mail address: getinfo@haworth.com].

The contracture of the muscle causes the head to tilt toward the side of the tumor with the chin rotated contralaterally. The tumor persists for 2 to 3 months and gradually disappears at about 4 to 6 months of age.[1] Plagiocephaly, craniofacial asymmetry, scoliosis, shortening of other neck structures (trapezius, scalene and platysma muscles and the carotid sheath), and delayed motor development may be identified along with persistence or progression of SCM contracture.[1-5]

ASSESSMENT

The purpose of this article is to present a systematic approach to the assessment and conservative treatment of the patient with torticollis. Assessment begins with acquisition of past medical history. We use the assessment form in Figure 1. Information collected includes birth history, other medical problems, diagnosis, and diagnostic test results. Personal/social skills, behavioral responses, and respiratory status can be observed throughout the assessment.

Postural Patterns and Range of Motion

The next step is to identify whether the patient has a left or right torticollis. A contracture of the right SCM muscle produces a right torticollis with the face turned toward the left and the top of the head tilted toward the right.[6] The left SCM is elongated and weak and cervical scoliosis is convex toward the left.[6] Shortening of the right upper trapezius and left splenius capitis muscles may also be present. The opposite pattern is observed in a left torticollis.[6] Muscular torticollis appears to be more common on the right side.[7-9]

The SCM muscle should be palpated on both sides of the neck from origin to insertion and findings of a fibrotic nodule, diffuse fibrosis, or normal muscle tissue tension and elasticity should be recorded. The severity and distribution of fibrosis differ from patient to patient. The fibrotic tumor is a hard, painless swelling, 1-3 cm. in diameter, within the substance of the muscle. It may develop between 14 and 21 days after birth and be undetectable by palpation by age 6 months.[1]

Secondary shortening may be observed in the trunk muscles with a convexity ipsilateral or contralateral to the involved side. Total

FIGURE 1. Torticollis assessment form pages 1-5. Pages 1-3 provide for recording of assessment results. Page 4 summarizes problems noted, and page 5 outlines the goals and treatment plan.

Patient name: _____

Torticollis Evaluation Form

Hospital number: _____

☐ Inpatient   ☐ Outpatient

D.O.B.: _____

Date:_____ Chronological age: _____ Referral Source: _____
Age at onset:_____ Age at diagnosis:_____ Race:_____ Sex:_____
Pediatrician/family physician: _____ Orthopedic Surgeon: _____
Torticollis: ☐ left   ☐ right
X-rays: ☐ cervical   -   ☐ hip   ☐ spine   ☐ other: _____
             ☐ comment: _____
Social/family history: _____

Pregnancy/labor/
delivery complications: _____
Delivery: ☐ c-section   ☐ vaginal   ☐ breech   ☐ suction   ☐ forceps   ☐ nuchal cord
             ☐ twin A   ☐ twin B   ☐ other:_____
Birth weight:_____ Birth order:_____ Weeks gestation: _____ Apgars:_____
Hip status: ☐ WNL   ☐ dislocated ☐ dysplastic ☐ left   ☐ right
Feeding: ☐ bottle   ☐ nursing   feeding problems: _____
Related problems/diagnoses:_____

Ocular exam: _____
Palpation SCM: ☐ nl   ☐ diffuse fibrosis
             ☐ fibrotic mass specify: ☐ left   ☐ right   mass size: _____
Craniofacial asymmetry: ☐ mild   ☐ moderate ☐ severe
Plagiocephaly: ☐ mild   ☐ moderate ☐ severe   ☐ concordant ☐ discordant
Hemihypoplasia: ☐ mild   ☐ moderate ☐ severe
Typical posture: supine _____
                             prone _____
                             sit _____
                             stand _____
                             transitions _____
Behavior: ☐ tolerates handling   ☐ irritable with handling
Respiratory:
             ☐ WNL   ☐ retractions ☐ nasal flare ☐ changes with activity
             ☐ other: _____
Skin: _____
Visual:
             Focus on objects ☐ yes   ☐ no
             Visual pursuit   ☐ left   ☐ right   ☐ up   ☐ down   ☐ diagonal
                               ☐ peripheral
             Test positions   ☐ head tilt L ☐ head tilt R ☐ head held in midline   ☐ supine
                               ☐ supported sit   ☐ independent sit
Developmental Test Used and Results:_____

Therapist's initials:

Page 1

FIGURE 1 (continued)

Patient name: _____
Hospital number: _____

Joint Evaluation/ROM

Passive tested supine:

Neck	_____ degrees flexion	_____	degrees extension
Neck lateral flexion	_____ degrees left	_____	degrees right
Neck rotation	_____ degrees left	_____	degrees right
Active rotation supine:	_____ degrees left	_____	degrees right
Active rotation sit:	_____ degrees left	_____	degrees right
Active rotation prone:	_____ degrees left	_____	degrees right
Active rotation stand:	_____ degrees left	_____	degrees right

UE's: ☐ no limitations   ☐ limitations: _____

LE's: ☐ no limitations   ☐ limitations: _____

Trunk: ☐ no limitations   ☐ limitations: _____

Muscle Tone

UE's: ☐ hypo   ☐ low   ☐ nl   ☐ high   ☐ hyper
     ☐ unable to assess, describe: _____

LE's: ☐ hypo   ☐ low   ☐ nl   ☐ high   ☐ hyper
     ☐ unable to assess, describe: _____

Trunk: ☐ hypo   ☐ low   ☐ nl   ☐ high   ☐ hyper
     ☐ unable to assess, describe: _____

Neck: ☐ hypo   ☐ low   ☐ nl   ☐ high   ☐ hyper
     ☐ unable to assess, describe: _____

Strength

	Full movement against gravity	Partial movement against gravity	No movement against gravity	Not assessed	Test position
Neck flexion					
Neck extension					
Neck lateral flexion Left					
Neck lateral flexion Right					
Neck rotation Left					
Neck rotation Right					
Trunk flexion					
Trunk extension					
Trunk lateral flexion Left					
Trunk lateral flexion Right					
Left Upper Extremity					
Right Upper Extremity					
Left Lower Extremity					
Right Lower Extremity					
Other strength tests:					

Pull-to-sit:

Head tilt
☐ yes
☐ no
___ deg.

Head lag
☐ yes
☐ no
___ deg.

Trunk tilt
☐ yes
☐ no

Therapist's initials:

_____
Page 2

Postural Reactions

Patient name:_____

Hospital number:_____

<u>Vertical Neck Righting</u>

Upright tilt 45° (2.5-6 mo.):

full response	☐ L	☐ R
partial response	☐ L	☐ R
no response	☐ L	☐ R
not assessed	☐ L	☐ R

Upright tilt anterior dir. 45° (2.5-6 mo.):

full response	☐ L	☐ R
partial response	☐ L	☐ R
no response	☐ L	☐ R
not assessed	☐ L	☐ R

Upright tilt posterior dir. 45° (2.5-6 mo.):

full response	☐ L	☐ R
partial response	☐ L	☐ R
no response	☐ L	☐ R
not assessed	☐ L	☐ R

Prone (1.5-4 mo.):

full response	☐ L	☐ R
partial response	☐ L	☐ R
no response	☐ L	⊓ R
not assessed	☐ L	☐ R

Supine (5 mo.):

full response	☐ L	☐ R
partial response	☐ L	☐ R
no response	☐ L	☐ R
not assessed	☐ L	☐ R

<u>Rotational Righting Reaction (6-12 mo.):</u>

full response	☐ L	☐ R
partial response	☐ L	☐ R
no response	☐ L	☐ R
not assessed	☐ L	☐ R

<u>Protective Extension Reactions</u>

Downward (6-7 mo.):

full response	☐ L	☐ R
partial response	☐ L	☐ R
no response	☐ L	☐ R
not assessed	☐ L	☐ R

Forward (6-9 mo.):

full response	☐ L	☐ R
partial response	☐ L	☐ R
no response	☐ L	☐ R
not assessed	☐ L	☐ R

Sideways (6-11 mo.):

full response	☐ L	☐ R
partial response	☐ L	☐ R
no response	☐ L	☐ R
not assessed	☐ L	☐ R

Backward (9-12 mo.):

full response	☐ L	☐ R
partial response	☐ L	☐ R
no response	☐ L	☐ R
not assessed	☐ L	☐ R

Therapist's initials:

FIGURE 1 (continued)

Postural Reactions (continued)

Patient name: _____
Hospital number: _____

<u>Equilibrium Reactions</u>

Prone (5-9 mo.):

full response	☐ L	☐ R
partial response	☐ L	☐ R
no response	☐ L	☐ R
not assessed	☐ L	☐ R

Supine (7-11 mo.):

full response	☐ L	☐ R
partial response	☐ L	☐ R
no response	☐ L	☐ R
not assessed	☐ L	☐ R

Sitting (7-8 mo.):

full response	☐ L	☐ R
partial response	☐ L	☐ R
no response	☐ L	☐ R
not assessed	☐ L	☐ R

Quadruped (8-12 mo.):

full response	☐ L	☐ R
partial response	☐ L	☐ R
no response	☐ L	☐ R
not assessed	☐ L	☐ R

Standing (12-21 mo.):

full response	☐ L	☐ R
partial response	☐ L	☐ R
no response	☐ L	☐ R
not assessed	☐ L	☐ R

Other Reflex Tests: _____

Assessment Problems

☐ Torticollis: ☐ L   ☐ R   ☐ mild   ☐ moderate   ☐ severe
     ☐ plagiocephaly   ☐ hemihypoplasia

☐ Decreased neck passive range of motion:

☐ lateral flexion L	☐ rotation L
☐ lateral flexion R	☐ rotation R
☐ flexion	☐ extension

☐ Decreased trunk passive range of motion:

☐ lateral flexion L	☐ rotation L
☐ lateral flexion R	☐ rotation R
☐ flexion	☐ extension

☐ Decreased strength: ☐ neck   ☐ trunk   ☐ UE's   ☐ LE's
☐ Decreased active neck rotation: ☐ L   ☐ R   ☐ supine   ☐ prone
     ☐ sit   ☐ stand
☐ No midline head-to-trunk cntrl: ☐ supine   ☐ prone   ☐ sit   ☐ stand
☐ No visual tracking: ☐ L   ☐ R   ☐ up   ☐ down
     ☐ diagonal ☐ peripheral
☐ Postural alignment problems
☐ Vestibular and/or sensory problems
☐ Head righting responses: ☐ no response   ☐ L   ☐ R
     ☐ partial response   ☐ L   ☐ R
☐ Equilibrium responses: ☐ no response   ☐ L   ☐ R
     ☐ partial response   ☐ L   ☐ R
☐ Development delay: _____
☐ Other: _____

Therapist's initials:

Page 4

Rehabilitation Potential   □ poor   □ fair   Patient name:_____
   □ good   □ excellent   Hospital number:_____

Goals
   Short term time frame:_____
   Short term goals:_____
_____
_____
_____
_____
_____
_____

   Long term time frame:_____
   Long term goals:_____
_____
_____
_____
_____
_____
_____

Treatment Plan
   Frequency of treatment:_____
   Duration of treatment:_____

    □ Neck ROM   □ Bracing   □ TOT   □ Foam
    □ Trunk ROM   □ Development exercises   collar
    □ Extremity ROM   □ Manual therapy
    □ Positioning devices   □ Parent education/home program
    □ Strength exercises   □ SI intervention
    □ Positioning/handling   □ Postural education exercises
      techniques
    □ Other:_____
_____
_____
_____
_____

Referral Recommendations
    □ OT/PT
    □ Orthopedics
    □ Pediatric Surgery
    □ Plastic Surgery
    □ Pediatric Neurology
    □ Pediatric Neurosurgery
    □ Opthalmology

_____
Therapist's signature and date
Phone number:_____
Fax number:_____

Page 5

spinal misalignment, or scoliosis, may occur as a result of the muscle imbalance.[1,3,10] Ruedemann, in a series of case studies, illustrated the scoliosis produced when weakness of the longitudinal spinal muscles is present from birth.[10]

In torticollis posture, the fascial system compensates for the body's asymmetric posturing in one of two ways; involuntary compensation for SCM torticollis may occur by elevation of the shoulder on the affected side (Figure 2) or by a lateral shift of the head toward the affected side (Figure 3).[1] The authors' clinical observations of posture suggest that a laterally flexed head causes a shift in the center of mass, and the whole upper body laterally shifts to re-establish the midline balance. These adjustments result in small curves at the cervical and lumbar spine, constant tension on the lower back muscles, a tilted shoulder girdle axis, and broadening of the shoulder on the non-involved side.

During assessment, one must consider whether other soft tissue structures are affected, locate any compensatory restrictions, and evaluate how these impairments affect the overall ability to perform motor functions. Functionally, the adult cervical spine can allow movements of 160-180 degrees total rotation, 90 degrees total lateral flexion, and 130 degrees total flexion and extension.[11] Numerous muscles are concerned with movements of the head and the neck. The SCM muscle has an origin attachment at two heads: one head from the upper border of the manubrium sterni, partly covering the sternoclavicular joint, and the other from the upper, medial third of the border of the clavicle.[6] The insertion is on the mastoid process of the temporal bone and the lateral half of the superior nuchal line of the occipital bone.[6] The SCM muscles are innervated by the accessory nerve[6] and act bilaterally to extend and flex the head and neck. Unilateral action laterally flexes the head toward the ipsilateral shoulder and rotates it to point the chin cranially and to the opposite side.[6] SCM muscle action raises the thorax when the head is fixed.[6] The trapezius muscle acts as a synergist of the ipsilateral SCM muscle and is also innervated by the accessory nerve.[6] Other lateral flexors of the cervical spine include the scalenes, the longissimus capitis, rectus capitis lateralis, longus coli, obliquus capitis, splenius capitis, and intertransversarii muscles.[6] The suboccipital muscles collectively function in the actions of extension, lateral flexion and rotation of the head.[6]

FIGURE 2. A diagram showing spontaneous involuntary compensation for torticollis by elevation of the shoulder on the affected side. Compensatory posture leads to head alignment perpendicular to the support surface. (Acknowledgment for Figure 2—From Jones PG. *Torticollis in Infancy and Childhood,* 1968. Courtesy of Charles C Thomas, Publisher, Springfield, Illinois.)

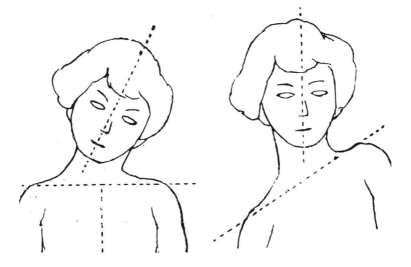

FIGURE 3. A diagram showing compensation for torticollis by the production of cervical scoliosis with two curves. (Acknowledgment for Figure 3—From Jones PG. *Torticollis in Infancy and Childhood,* 1968. Courtesy of Charles C Thomas, Publisher, Springfield, Illinois.)

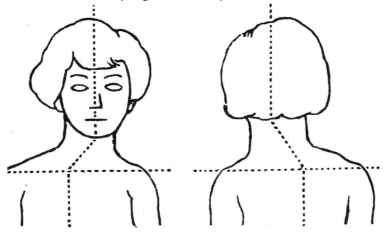

The need to evaluate the entire musculoskeletal system cannot be over-emphasized. Fascial interconnections can be traced from the top of the cranium down the entire body and into the foot.[12] Key areas to check for restriction in the presence of torticollis are the SCM and lateral cervical muscles in addition to the platysma,[13] pectoralis major and minor and their attachments into the upper arm and scapula, biceps brachia, wrist flexor and pronator muscles. Further down the trunk, evaluation of the ipsilateral quadratus lumborum attachments from the twelfth rib into the iliac crest should occur, followed by the hip rotators and the iliotibial tract into the calf musculature. Segmental motion testing of the spine at transitional areas, occiput-C_1, C_7-T_1, and L_5-S_1 should also be checked. Rib function must be checked for restrictions which can exist in either inhalation or exhalation movements. Children with torticollis posture should have their craniosacral systems evaluated for restrictions. We find the most common areas for cranial restrictions to be the temporal bones. We believe this finding to be due in large part to limitation caused by the SCM muscle where it attaches to the mastoid process of the temporal bone.

It is important to rule out ocular torticollis as a cause for head tilt. The head tilt in ocular torticollis is a response to an imbalance of the extraocular muscles.[3,10,14] In cases of ocular torticollis, the occlusion of one eye will normally allow the head to straighten.[3,14] A positive sit-up test for ocular torticollis is one in which the head tilt observed in a sitting position resolves when the patient is in a supine position.[14] Patients with long-standing ocular torticollis may, however, develop secondary contracture of the SCM muscle and present with a false-negative sit-up test.[14]

Both congenital muscular torticollis and uncorrected vertical facial asymmetry can cause a difference in height of the eyes and an abnormal head position.[3,15] A postural change of the spine and its musculature will develop as the infant places visual demands to achieve binocularity by compensating to level the eyes.[3,15] Binocular fusion develops by the fifth or sixth month of life.[3] To maintain binocularity during precise active vision, a tilting of the head may occur to level or equalize the heights of the eyes.[3,14]

Vision is the dominant information-gathering system and the body will make many adaptations to maintain the system.[3] Visual pursuit skills should be assessed in all developmentally appropriate postures. Vision should be assessed both with and without correction of head alignment. It is important to observe the head tilt posture during dynamic, static, and passive vision. During dynamic vision (vision used while in motion), binocular vision is loosely maintained, allowing the head to remain vertical for tasks of walking and climbing.[3] On the other hand, both static vision, which requires eye movement while position of the body changes little (lateral pursuit movements) and passive vision, in which there is no body motion and little eye movement (viewing television, staring), demand a high level of binocularity.[3] These differences in use of the visual system during different tasks may in part explain why the child continues to have an intermittent head tilt even after range of motion and strength have been restored.[3]

Skeletal Asymmetry

Another secondary impairment associated with torticollis is plagiocephaly (from Greek, translated as "twisted skull").[1] Plagiocephaly is a persistent molding of the fetal head with a positional etiology or resulting from unilateral closure of the coronal or lambdoid suture (Figure 4).[1,3] Craniosynostosis that occurs unilaterally significantly limits growth in the stenosed area. The difference in the rate of growth between the two sides of the skull produces a bulge on the normal side and a flattened area on the affected side (concordant).[1] Various terms are used to describe the most common abnormal headshapes caused by craniosynostosis.[16,17]

Jones hypothesized that the postnatal development of plagiocephaly in infants with torticollis occurred as a result of deforming forces caused by constant contact of the head with the resting surface with little or no variation in the position of the head.[1] In the supine position, the hemi-occiput on the side opposite the affected muscle becomes the area which most often bears the weight of the cranium. Clinically, one may observe an arrest of the plagiocephaly at the age of four to six months when the infant can sit up, and range of motion in the neck muscles is improved. The type of facial asymmetry that occurs as a result of torticollis is best described as hemihypoplasia.[1] On the side of the affected muscle, the contour of the cheek is flattened, and the vertical height of the face is diminished while the horizontal width is usually greater than that of the contralateral side (Figure 5).[1] Classical plagiocephaly, on the other

FIGURE 4A. Diagram of plagiocephaly as seen from the vertex (norma verticalis). The left frontal and right occipital regions are prominent, while there is relative flattening of the diagonally opposite regions. The long axis of the ellipse (P) is deflected from the sagittal plane to the left; *b* is longer than *a*, reflecting the greater width of the right half of the face when viewed from the front. (Acknowlegment for Figure 4A–From Jones PG. *Torticollis in Infancy and Childhood,* 1968. Courtesy of Charles C Thomas, Publisher, Springfield, Illinois.)

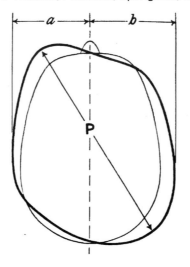

FIGURE 4B. Photographs demonstrating how the pinna on the side of the flattened occiput (a) is folded forwards (b), during rotation of the head, by contact with the surface on which the head lies in the supine position. (Acknowledgment for Figure 4B–From Jones PG. *Torticollis in Infancy and Childhood,* 1968. Courtesy of Charles C Thomas, Publisher, Springfield, Illinois.)

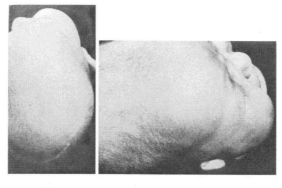

(a)   (b)

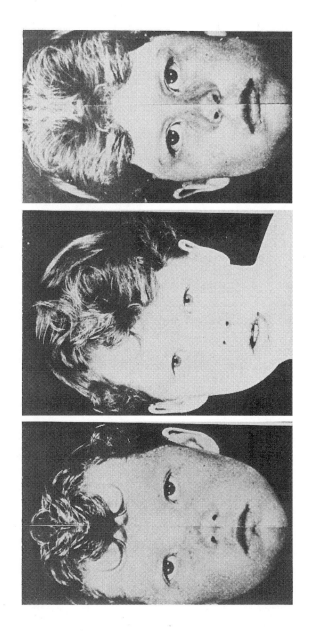

FIGURE 5. Facial asymmetry. Frontal photograph divided along the median plane and reprocessed, each side being paired with its mirror image, yielding two slightly different faces. (Acknowledgment for Figure 5–From Jones PG. *Torticollis in Infancy and Childhood*, 1968. Courtesy of Charles C Thomas, Publisher, Springfield, Illinois.)

hand, involves some asymmetry of the face in the horizontal dimension, but lacks the decreased vertical dimension of hemihypoplasia.[1]

Coventry and Harris, based on their series of 35 infants with SCM muscle tumor, reported that craniofacial asymmetry appeared at about four months, reached its peak at ten months, and had usually disappeared at fourteen months of age.[18] Facial asymmetry with a curvature in relation to the vertical axis is termed facial scoliosis.[19,20]

A patient who presents with or has a developing facial hemihypoplasia should be referred for surgical intervention. Facial hemihypoplasia has been found to develop in patients in whom torticollis persisted beyond the age of six months.[1] Hemihypoplasia may be absent when both SCM muscles are affected, and hemihypoplasia can develop following torticollis even when there is no SCM muscle fibrosis and no tension in this muscle.[1] In addition to facial hemihypoplasia, other criteria for surgical intervention may include:[21]

1. Persistence of an intramuscular tumor.
2. An increased thickening of the SCM muscle at six months of age.
3. Range of passive rotation persistently reduced by 30 degrees or more for a four-week interval after six months of age.
4. An increase in the deformity.
5. Persistence of the deformity after the age of twelve months.

Typical head and trunk posture should be observed in all positions. The patient should be undressed so that the clinician can observe head and body alignment relative to a line perpendicular to the support surface and ability to center the head relative to the midline of the trunk in a supine position. Supine head centering is normative in either preterm or full term infants at about 15 weeks past term.[22]

Cervical spine range of motion (ROM) should be measured for both passive and active range in a variety of positions. A safe, easy, and accurate way to measure cervical spinal motion for rotation, lateral flexion, and angle of head tilt is to use a universal goniometer that has been adapted with two carpenter's levels attached to its stationary arm. One level is located parallel to the stationary arm of the goniometer along its midline, and the other level is positioned perpendicular to the first level at the end of the goniometer's stationary arm[23] (Figure 6).

The patient is placed in supine with their head off the end of the plinth. The therapist should hold the patient supine against the plinth and keep the shoulders from elevating. The patient's head is centered and rotated. Neck rotation is the angle measured between the sagittal plane of the trunk (the stationary arm of the goniometer is placed in this plane at the top of the patient's head using the carpenter's level which is perpendicular to the midline of the goniometer's stationary arm) and the sagittal plane of the head at the end of the passive rotation (the movable arm of the goniometer is aligned with the nose of the infant–Figure 7a).[23] Infants may have 100 to 120 degrees of neck rotation to either side.[23] Rotation in sitting can also be assessed using the modified goniometer (Figure 7b).

FIGURE 6. Range of motion measurement of lateral flexion of the head in supine.

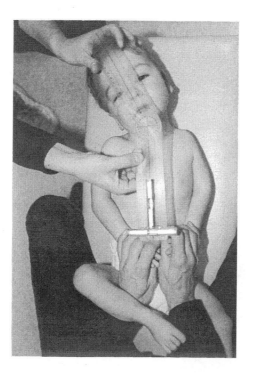

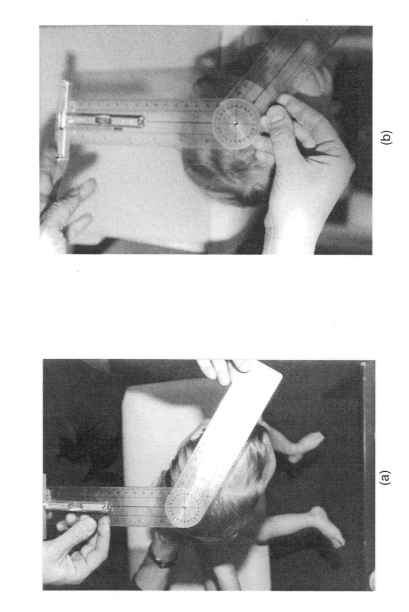

FIGURE 7. Range of motion measurement of neck rotation in (a) supine and (b) sitting.

Lateral neck flexion should be measured in supine (Figure 6) and in supported or independent sitting position (Figure 8). The stationary arm of the goniometer can be maintained horizontal by leveling the carpenter's bubble and the moveable arm can be aligned with the lateral corner of the child's eye.[23] Eliciting head righting responses to measure active lateral neck flexion may be accomplished by using an adapted car seat that can rotate on a hinge with angle degrees behind the chair while the patient wears a cervical range of motion (CROM) device (CROM, Performance Attainment Associates, 958 Lydia Drive, Roseville, MN 55113) (Figure 9).[24] The CROM device is designed to measure cervical ROM in all three cardinal planes of motion without manual adjustment.[24] The CROM device is aligned on the nose bridge and ears and fastened to the head by a

FIGURE 8. Range of motion measurement of lateral flexion in sitting.

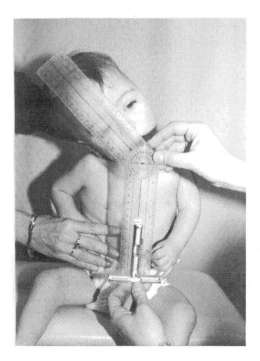

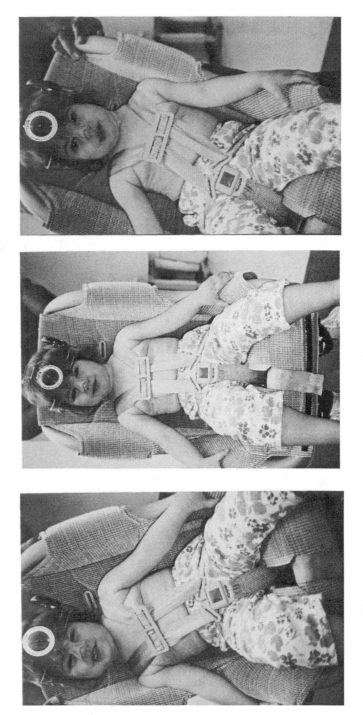

FIGURE 9. Documenting range of head movement by eliciting lateral head righting responses in tilt chair using a CROM device on a 20-month-old child with left torticollis upon (a) 45-degree tilt right, (b) vertical chair alignment, and (c) 45-degree tilt left.

(a)   (b)   (c)

Velcro strap.[24] The CROM device may also be used to measure lateral flexion of the head in sitting and other postures.

Motor Performance

The development of early motor skills may be influenced by presence of torticollis posture. Factors such as muscle tone, an imbalance in muscle strength, abnormal postural patterns, lack of cervical mobility, and secondary fascial restrictions may delay acquisition of skills such as turning the head toward the involved side, upper extremity reaching on the ipsilateral side, weight-shifting of the trunk, rolling, prone propping on elbows, crawling, sitting, and an assortment of transitional movements from one posture to another. Binder and associates reported in a retrospective review of 277 children with CMT that immobility in the cervical area often leads to stiffness in the trunk and asymmetrical motor development.[2]

Several developmental tests can be used to document posture and control of movement for function. The Test of Infant Motor Performance (TIMP) may prove to be a good test for infants with torticollis posture because a major construct assessed is the infant's ability independently to control head position in a variety of spatial orientations.[25] The clinician should choose developmental tests that include items of head control, head and trunk posture, reflexes, righting reactions, postural tone, flexibility, strength, and gross and fine motor skills. Other test possibilities are:

- INFANIB: Infant Neurological International Battery[26]
- The Peabody Developmental Motor Scales (PDMS)[27]
- The Movement Assessment of Infants (MAI)[28]
- The Bayley II[29]

Spontaneous movements involving neck rotation are assessed as the child lies in supine and prone and in supported or independent sitting and standing, depending on age and abilities. The lengthening capacity (extensibility) of the trapezius muscles can be evaluated by observing the speed of shoulder elevation when the arms are pulled down and then released. The three components of muscle tone–consistency, extensibility, and passivity–can also be checked in the muscles of the extremities and trunk.[28,30]

The patient's ability to change positions, isolate requested movements, lift the head off supporting surfaces in supine, prone, and sidelying, or demonstrate graded control and adaptive responses is dependent on muscle strength. Strength can be estimated by observing active movement in a variety of positions both pro- and anti-gravity. Gross strength may be graded as full, partial, or no movement with test position identified to indicate whether the patient was in a pro- or anti-gravity position (Figure 1, page 2).

Assessment of postural reactions includes evaluation of three groups of responses: righting reactions, protective reactions, and equilibrium reactions (Figure 1, pages 3, 4). Grading of responses is based on completeness of the reaction. For example, alignment of the head to vertical with the mouth horizontal is a complete response in a righting reaction. Restoration of the body parts to normal alignment following rotation of some body segment is a complete response for rotational righting reactions. Extension of the upper extremities in the same general direction of a displacing force which shifts the body's center of gravity is the full response for protective reactions. Finally, changes of posture or movement which seek to restore disturbed balance when the body's base of support is shifted, either due to a push, pull, or tilt, is the full response for equilibrium reactions.[31] Remember while observing responses to watch for the patient's ability to bring the head past midline toward the uninvolved side and for the appropriate pattern and sequence of movement (Figure 10).

The vestibulocolic and cervicocolic reflexes and the viscoelastic properties of the neck muscles all contribute to appropriate, coordinated neck muscle activity to stabilize the head in space and in relation to the body.[32,33] Diminished response in the lengthened SCM muscle caused by the increased head-neck angle in the frontal, transverse, and sagittal planes affects muscle performance of both the neck and the trunk.[32,33] Asymmetries in postural responses should be noted during evaluation.

Typically, patients with torticollis posture may be unable to right the head laterally toward the uninvolved side and may over-react when righting the head toward the involved side. Trunk response in postural reactions may also be absent on the uninvolved side (Figure 11). The patient may have difficulty with actively rotating their head toward the involved side (Figure 12). The authors' clinical observations of the sequence of return of strength and movement of the overstretched uninvolved side is first in the trunk, then neck muscles, followed by a reversal in sequencing of the reaction to head and neck first and then trunk.

An infant or child with torticollis may have more than one deformity. Various combinations of torticollis, plagiocephaly, scoliosis and thoracic asymmetry will effect the ability to weight shift using postural reactions. As an example, the progression for an infant or child with a left torticollis and a c-curve scoliosis on the side of the neck convexity (non-involved side) from most difficult to least difficult combinations of trunk and neck rotation with lateral flexion, extension, and flexion would be:

1. Trunk: left rotation, right lateral flexion, extension;
   Neck: left rotation, right lateral flexion, extension
2. Trunk: right rotation, right lateral flexion, flexion;
   Neck: right rotation, right lateral flexion, flexion
3. Trunk: left rotation, left lateral flexion, flexion;
   Neck: left rotation, left lateral flexion, flexion
4. Trunk: right rotation, left lateral flexion, extension;
   Neck: right rotation, left lateral flexion, extension.

The ability to use diagonal patterns in the transverse plane (rotation) depends upon the development of movement control in the saggittal plane (extension and flexion) and movement control in the frontal plane (lateral flexion). Movement control of rotation with extension develops before rotation with flexion, extension develops before flexion, and lateral flexion develops after extension and flexion. The spinal restrictions and muscular imbalances of a left torticollis will cause: (1) a lack of extension and rotation in the thoracic spine, (2) a limit in expansion of the left shoulder girdle for retraction, and (3) a change of concentric and eccentric control of the neck and trunk muscles. The cervical spine will lack varying degrees of joint motion including right cervical facet side bending and left gliding.

Based on evaluation of the assessment results, a list of problems can be identified, and short and long-term goals can be established (Figure 1, pages 4, 5). Other appropriate referral recommendations can also be indicated on the assessment form (Figure 1, page 5).

TREATMENT

Emery (this volume) reviews outcomes addressed in the clinical research literature. Selection of appropriate treatment techniques

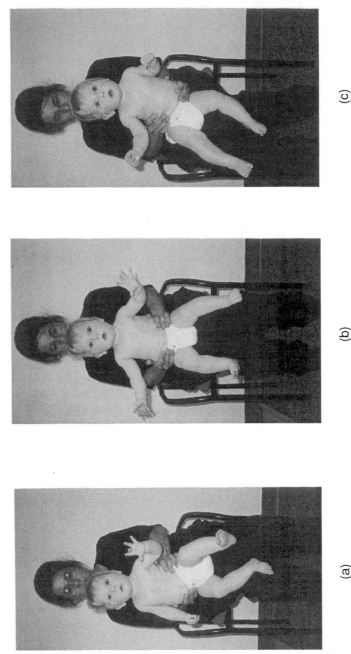

FIGURE 10. Postural reactions of a 5-month-old infant with right torticollis to (a) sitting tilt right, (b) sitting midline, (c) sitting tilt left, (d) vertical suspension tilt right, (e) vertical suspension midline, (f) vertical tilt left. There is no change in head to trunk alignment with righting response to the left (non-involved side) versus over-reaction to the right (involved side). There is less trunk response to the non-involved side in vertical suspension versus sitting when pelvis is stabilized on a surface.

(a)   (b)   (c)

42

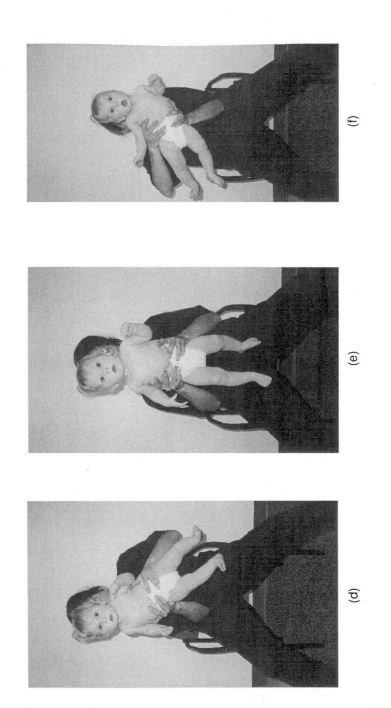

(d)

(e)

(f)

43

44

FIGURE 11. Six-month-old infant with left torticollis during (a) vertical suspension tilt 45 degrees right, (b) vertical suspension midline with habitual left head tilt, (c) vertical suspension tilt 45 degrees left, (d) vertical suspension tilt 90 degrees right, (e) vertical suspension tilt 90 degrees left, (f) head righting sidelying right, (g) head righting sidelying left. Responses when tilted toward the left or lying on the left side are incomplete.

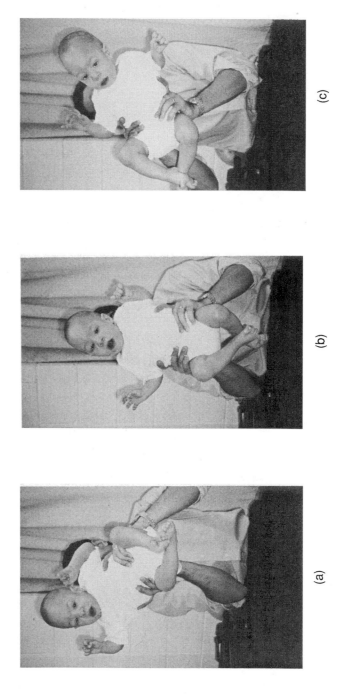

(a)

(b)

(c)

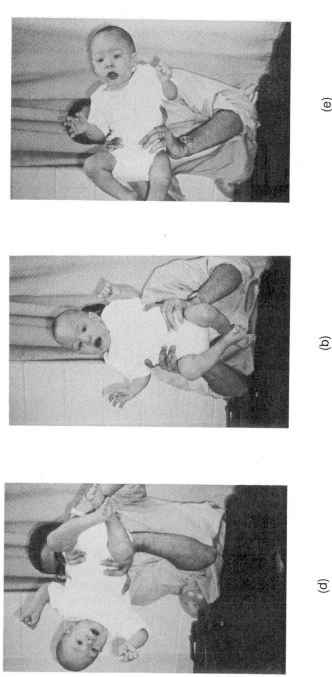

(e)

(b)

(d)

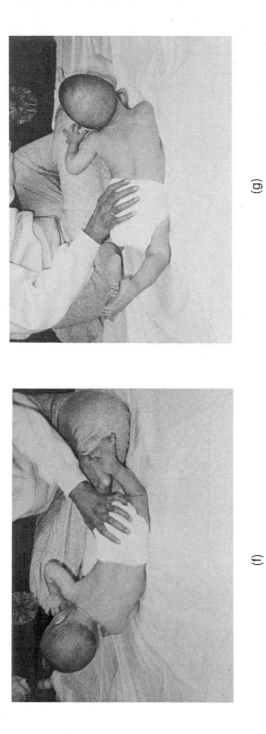

FIGURE 11 (continued)

(g)

(f)

will depend on the goals established on the basis of the assessment results and on the age of the patient (Table 1). For most children, however, treatment considerations include management of muscle hypoextensibility and strength, positioning and handling instructions, and postural education. These areas of management are discussed in the following sections, along with frequency and duration of treatment and anticipated outcomes. Table 2 describes the typical protocol for the first four visits.

Muscle Hypoextensibility

At the initial visit, parents and other caretakers are instructed in stretching the involved SCM, upper trapezius, and ipsilateral trunk muscles and provided with written instructions for a home program (Figure 13). Two people may be required to stretch the infant's neck. One person secures the patient's shoulders, stabilizing the clavicles, while the other person aligns the head in midline and rotates or laterally flexes the head to stretch the affected muscles. Slight traction, massage and warm compresses may be used to relax the muscle prior to stretching (Figure 14). Two periods of stretching daily, in which each stretch of rotation and lateral flexion of the neck is repeated five times holding each stretch for 10 seconds, was found successful in gaining normal range-of-motion of the neck after a mean treatment duration of 4.7 months.[23] In long-standing cases of torticollis, shortening of other neck structures may occur, including the trapezius, scalene and platysma muscles and the carotid sheath.[4,13] Fine tuning the neck stretching exercises will be important in order to elongate all of the involved musculature. We use manual therapy, including soft tissue mobilization, joint mobilization, and craniosacral techniques to address joint and fascial system restrictions and asymmetries, always treating the most involved area first (Table 3).

During the course of treatment, it is important to alert the parents to the potential for regression of the torticollis posture and provide instructions for adapting the home program when changes occur. A child may lose ROM of the SCM muscle during a growth spurt because the SCM on the involved side does not grow at the same rate as the muscle on the uninvolved side.[7] In this case, parents should increase the time devoted to ROM exercises. The child may also lose active midline head control during periods of illness, teeth-

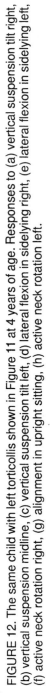

FIGURE 12. The same child with left torticollis shown in Figure 11 at 4 years of age. Responses to (a) vertical suspension tilt right, (b) vertical suspension midline, (c) vertical suspension tilt left, (d) lateral flexion in sidelying right, (e) lateral flexion in sidelying left, (f) active neck rotation right, (g) alignment in upright sitting, (h) active neck rotation left.

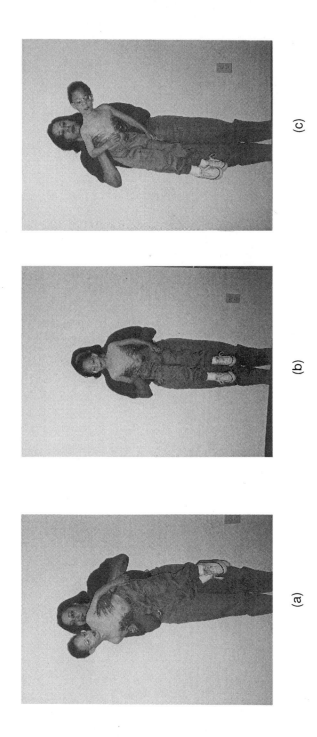

(a)

(b)

(c)

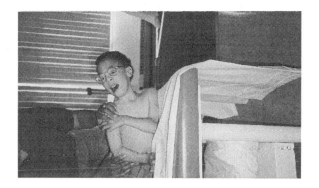

(e)

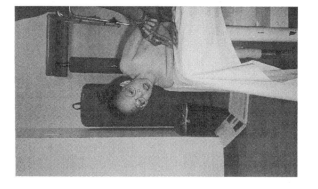

(d)

FIGURE 12 (continued)

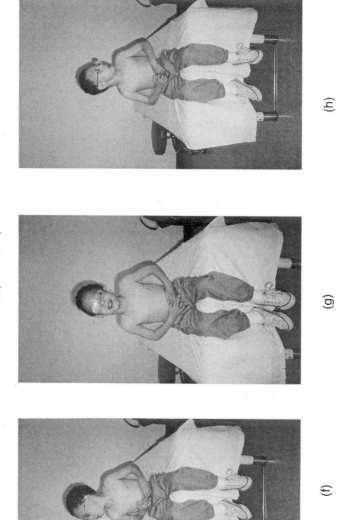

(f)

(g)

(h)

TABLE 1. Chronological Intervention Pathway for Muscular Torticollis

0-3 Months
1. Passive and active neck and trunk ROM
2. Strengthening exercises neck and trunk gravity assisted
3. Positioning and handling to promote midline and symmetry
4. Massage
5. Righting reactions supine, prone, sidelying
6. Postural education, opposite posture in supine while playing
7. Visual exercises to promote active head rotation toward the involved side
8. Environment adaptations to promote self-initiated functional movement patterns of head rotation toward the involved side, midline and symmetry
9. Developmental exercises as appropriate

4-5 Months
Everything listed 0-3 Months, plus:
1. Bracing
2. Righting and equilibrium reactions in supine, prone, sidelying, sitting and vertical suspension
3. Transitional movements and symmetrical weight-shifting skills
4. Shoulder girdle and trunk exercises
5. Symmetry in sacral-pelvic base
6. Eccentric neck and trunk strengthening
7. Specific concentric neck strengthening exercises:
   In prone—neck extension and asymmetrical neck extension
   In supine—neck flexion
   In sidelying—lateral neck flexion
8. Active head rotation in all postures

6-8 Months
Everything listed 0-5 Months, plus:
1. Righting and equilibrium reactions in quadruped
2. Protective extension reactions
3. Anti-gravity strengthening neck and trunk exercises

9-12 Months
Everything listed 0-8 Months, plus:
1. Upgrade balance and development exercises; equilibrium reactions in standing
2. Spread out visits and monitor as appropriate
3. Discontinue brace wear as appropriate

13-18 Months
Independent ambulator ready for discharge or 6-month interval follow-up. Parents can continue to work on strengthening endurance and normalizing equilibrium reaction sequences and timing. Home-based exercises as indicated to continue ROM, strength, endurance and postural control development. Developmental intervention as indicated.

TABLE 2. Torticollis Treatment Protocol

First Visit
Evaluation—musculoskeletal and developmental.
Home program
- passive neck stretches.
- positioning and handling to promote midline.
- environmental adaptations to promote self-initiated movements of head rotation toward involved side.

Second Visit
Reassess for ROM, strength and balance. Hands-on manual therapy with a focus on what caretakers found difficult in the home program. Ascertain what has gotten easy in the home program and how function has changed.
Home program
Review exercises and update home program to include exercises for:
- trunk elongation stretches.
- play in opposite posture in supine.
- toy placement and visual skills to promote active neck rotation and midline control.
- positioning to enhance head shape.

Third Visit
Reassess all equipment for positioning and observe parent handling, including lifting, carrying, placing and feeding. Hands-on manual therapy.
Home program
- repeat home program training from prior visits as needed.
- update program to include righting and equilibrium exercises to promote strength and postural control. Choice of exercises will be both age- and skill level-dependent.
- developmental exercises as indicated.

Fourth Visit
Continue to build repertoire of ROM, strengthening, development and postural education exercises. Note parent follow-through with ROM exercises, strength exercises, handling abilities and positioning skills. Always observe postural control and functional skills in all positions: supine, prone, sit, stand and transitions.
Home program
- home programs for strength, balance and development, and handling and positioning will require continued updating.

Subsequent Visits
Bracing of the neck: plan on one visit to fit the brace and let the parent(s) observe child wearing it for 30 minutes while engaged in parent-elicited play make sure that parents can don and doff the brace, understand how and when to use it, recognize vital sign changes if they occur with brace wear, and are comfortable with the child wearing the device.

FIGURE 13. Torticollis Exercise Sheets, pages 1, 2, 3.

Name: _____

ID #: _____

DOB: _____

Date: _____

TORTICOLLIS EXERCISES

Your child has a _____ torticollis. Their posture is _____ sidebent and _____ rotated.

STRETCHES: These stretches are to be done _____ daily, repeating the stretch _____ times, and holding the stretch for _____ counts. A good time to stretch is with diaper changes. Let your baby rest between each stretch. Do not persist if the baby resists. You may prepare the muscle to be stretched with gentle massage and/or warm compresses. Watch infant/child's face for changes in color, rate of breathing, eye rolling, perspiration or nasal flaring. Stop exercise if there are changes in any of these vital signs.

SIDEBEND STRETCH

_____ Left _____ Right

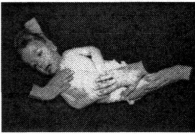

Head must be sidebent so ear touches shoulder.

– Place baby back/sitting/stomach/side.

– Positioned against floor/your chest/your legs.

– Hold down _____ shoulder with _____ hand.

– Sidebend head to _____ side with _____ hand.

Make sure chin and nose point straight up to the ceiling and the head is in midline to the trunk with a slight chin tuck during entire stretch movement. At the end of the sidebend movement you can introduce slight neck extension and/or flexion with the sidebend and rotation to the _____ side.

ROTATION STRETCH

_____ Left _____ Right

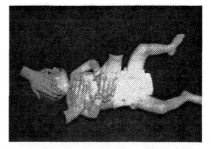

Head rotated so chin touches shoulder.

– Place baby back/sitting/stomach/side.

– Positioned against floor/your chest/your legs.

– Hold down _____ shoulder with _____ hand.

– Rotate head to _____ side with _____ hand.

Make sure chin and nose stay lined up and you start from a midline position with slight chin tuck. Maintain slight chin tuck through entire stretch movement. At the end of the rotation movement, you can introduce neck flexion and/or extension. Repeat starting position and rotate to the _____ side with chin tuck so that nose and mouth line up over _____ nipple to stretch back neck muscles on _____ side as you flex the head.

Therapist: _____

FIGURE 13 (continued)

Name: _____
ID #: _____
DOB: _____
Date: _____

TORTICOLLIS EXERCISES

Neck Rotation Stretch in Prone (on belly)

You can do the rotation stretch placing the child on
stomach and rotating head so face is to the_____ side.
The parent should cross his/her hands and hold the head
against the surface with one hand and the chest against
the surface with the other hand.

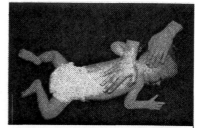

Trunk Stretch in Sidelying

Place child on_____ side so back is against your chest.
Place one hand at the hip and the other at_____ shoulder. Lift and pull hands away from each other. You can do
this stretch while standing or sitting and holding the infant.
A variation is to place the infant in sidelying so_____
shoulder is against your thigh and the head rests on top
of your thigh. You then lift the buttocks to stretch both
neck and trunk.

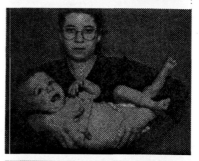

Trunk Stretch in Sitting

Sit with your hips and knees at a 90° angle and feet flat
on the floor. Place child straddled over your thigh. Spread
your hands and place your_____ hand over_____
ribs and_____ hand near_____ hip. Your_____
hand will move upward and_____ hand will move
downward as you shift the child to the side to elongate
_____ side of the trunk. Reverse hand placement
and repeat the stretch to the other side.

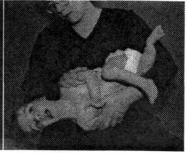

Place your hands spread on either side of the trunk. Move the child's trunk backwards to curve trunk into a
"C" and forward to extend/elongate trunk. Rotate the child's trunk by twisting it left and right keeping downward
pressure to hold child's buttocks onto your thigh. You may combine rotation with backward and forward
movement by moving the child diagonally as if drawing the letter "X" on your thigh with the child's trunk.

Repeat exercise_____ times_____ times a day.

Therapist:_____

Name: _____
ID #: _____
DOB: _____
Date: _____

TORTICOLLIS EXERCISES

Positioning

Place child on back (supine). Curve trunk to the _____ side, sidebend head _____ and rotate head to _____ side. Help the child hold this posture during play. Have the child play on back in this opposite position and also with head in midline to trunk.

To keep a midline head-to-trunk alignment in reclined sitting in a car seat, infant seat or swing, rolls should be used to support the child from head to hips on both sides.

Neck Strengthening in Play

During play lying on back (supine), lying on belly (prone), sitting supported or sitting independently, encourage _____ rotation and _____ sidebend of the head. In supported or independent sitting, keep the shoulders forward and do not let the shoulders twist as the child tries to rotate head to the _____ side. A good time to do this activity is while sitting in the high chair at mealtime. Visual stimulation or placement of toys can encourage head rotation. Use visual stimulation in all positions (back, side, stomach, sit, stand) to promote midline orientation and controlled head movement in all directions (up, down, sideways, diagonally, rotation). When presenting an item, hold it 8-12 inches from the infant's eyes.

Isolating Neck Muscle Activity

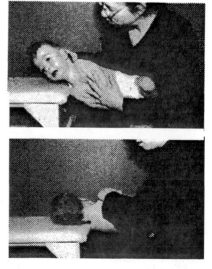

Strengthen the neck on _____ side by placing the child on _____ side over your thighs with head resting on another surface such as bed, couch or chair. Placing one arm and hand on child's _____ shouder/side/hip and your other hand at the head, help the child lift head off the surface using _____ neck muscles.

Repeat exercise _____ times, _____ times a day.

Therapist: _____

FIGURE 14. Neck passive range of motion exercises for child with right torticollis include (a) traction of posterior cervical neck muscles, (b) traction with flexion of posterior cervical neck muscles, (c) lateral neck flexion while stabilizing upper extremity, (d) lateral neck flexion stabilizing shoulder girdle and sternum, (e) neck rotation with extension, (f) neck rotation with flexion, (g) neck rotation in prone.

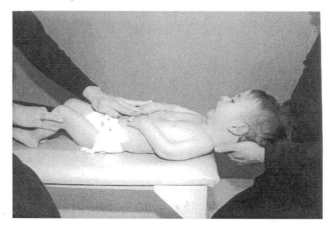

(a)

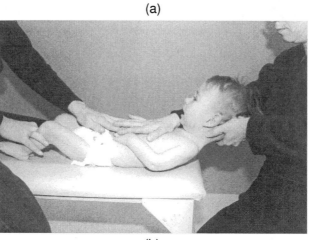

(b)

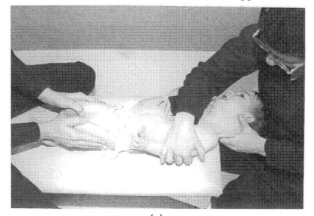

(c)

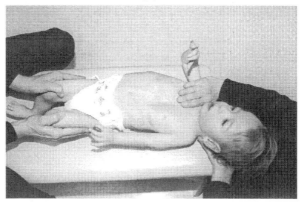

(d)

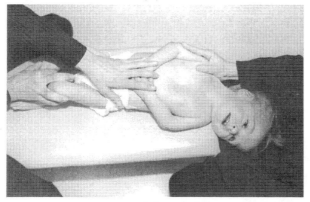

(e)

FIGURE 14 (continued)

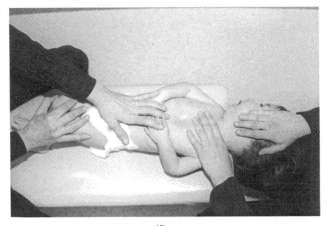

(f)

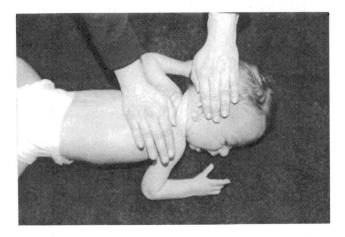

(g)

ing, or acquisition of new motor milestones. In this case, parents can devote increased attention to postural education exercises. The child should recover the previous level of head control and midline head postural alignment in 10-14 days. If not, a therapy visit may be needed for reassessment of the problem.

Davids and colleagues postulated that head position in utero can

TABLE 3. Manual Intervention Pathway for Muscular Torticollis

<u>Cranial/Cervical Area</u>
1. Soft tissue mobilization (massage, myofascial release techniques, etc.) to the anterior and posterior cervical musculature, with special attention to the SCM, suboccipitals and scalenes.
2. Mobilization of the cervical joints. Treat both convex and concave sides of the torticollis. Atlas/Axis as well as C6 and C7 are usually involved.
3. Craniosacral treatment with attention given to the temporal and splenoid bones. If plagiocephaly is present, all cranial sutures must be checked and treated.

<u>Thoracic/Shoulder</u>
1. Soft tissue mobilization to the anterior and posterior areas of the shoulder girdle including the subclavical, pectoralis minor, levator scapula, trapezius and respiratory diaphragm.
2. Mobilization of the shoulder complex, thoracic spine, scapula, sternum, ribs, and clavicle.

<u>Lumbar/Pelvis</u>
1. Soft tissue mobilization of the quadratus lumborum and hip rotators.
2. Mobilization techniques to the lumbar spine, the sacrum, and illia.

<u>Extremities</u>
1. Soft tissue mobilization to the upper extremities, especially the elbow extensors, forearm pronators, and wrist flexors.
2. Soft tissue mobilization of the lower extremities, especially the iliotibial band and calf musculature.

selectively injure the SCM muscle, leading to the development of intrauterine or perinatal compartment syndrome.[34] The mechanism of injury to the SCM muscle is localized "kinking" or "crush" caused by the position of the head and neck in utero or during labor and delivery.[34] The pathophysiology of the condition involves muscle ischemia, reperfusion, increased compartment pressure, edema, and neurological injury to the SCM muscle similar to what occurs in compartment syndrome of the leg or forearm.[34] Many infants with torticollis posture present as fussy, irritable babies with poor self-calming skills and low tolerance of positional changes and stimulation. They may react negatively to neck and trunk stretching. The infant presenting like this may also be recovering from the sequelae of an intrauterine or perinatal compartment syndrome and be experiencing pain.

Pain originating in the periphery is the result of noxious irritation of the nociceptors.[35] The nociceptors are activated by mechanical or chemical abnormalities in the tissues.[35] Throughout the human tissue there is a tridimensional plexus of unmyelinated fibers called the interstitial nociceptor system.[35] These receptors respond to excessive stretching or compression.[35] This system is also responsive to marked constriction or dilation of blood vessels.[35] The infant with congenital muscular torticollis could be responding to the sensory disturbances and experiencing pain as a result of a compartment syndrome.

Treatment modalities we have found useful with infants and children to relieve painful sensations are (1) superficial heat or cold, (2) massage, (3) accupressure, (4) vibration, (5) relaxation techniques and (6) hydrotherapy. The authors have found that using the sensory diet described by Wilbarger to be helpful.[36] This approach consists of infant massage, brushing, and gentle joint compression every two hours of the infant's awake time. Discomfort and irritable behavioral reactions during neck and trunk stretching exercise and during general therapeutic handling seem to be decreased.

Positioning and Handling

Therapeutic positioning and handling are addressed early in the intervention program. An initial goal of positioning is to develop midline postural control such that the head is in line with the body, the body is straight, the head is not tilted toward the involved side nor rotated away from the involved side, the chin is tucked, the arms are forward and down so that the hands can come together, and the legs are relaxed and together with hips flexed. Carrying the child can be used to help the child learn midline balance and body control. The parents can use their voices, visual contact, and their own (parents') body to encourage the child's control of head and body. For example, the child can be visually engaged as the parent holds him or her and moves about. With social interaction during the parent's movement, the child will experience vestibular stimulation and shifting of body weight as well as be distracted while the parent is placing the child in position of stretch or a more neutral postural alignment than the habitual abnormal posture. Whenever the child is placed into equipment such as the car seat, infant seat, or swing, dense foam inserts or rolls made of towels, diapers, or receiving blankets should be used to provide a midline position of postural alignment. The head and trunk should be supported on both sides. It is important to keep the pelvis level and avoid compensatory posturing of the trunk and pelvis when the head is prevented from laterally flexing.

Strength

Strengthening is begun with active-assistive movements of the head and trunk. Active head rotation is encouraged by placing toys on the involved side, and by talking to and feeding the patient from the involved side. The use of specific eccentric, concentric, and isometric strength exercises, the use of headband weights, or the use of biofeedback will depend on age and cooperation level of the patient and on interest and cooperation of the family or other caregivers (Figures 15, 16, 17, 18).

Postural Control

Postural education to promote symmetry and balanced muscle activity should address control of the body's position in space for stability and for orientation of the head to the trunk. The use of lateral head righting responses may begin at four months of age in upright, rolling and sidelying activities for strengthening and postural education (Figures 15, 16). All aspects of postural control processing should be considered and used as part of the treatment. The patient needs to have midline orientation and capacity for movement away from a midline orientation while: sustaining a posture, regaining a posture, moving between postures, exploring and manipulating objects, and locomoting. The postural control systems used to coordinate these motor behaviors include sensory (visual, vestibular, somatosensory), musculoskeletal (flexibility, strength, endurance), neuromuscular (timing and sequencing of muscle activation patterns), adaptive mechanisms, and anticipatory control processes.[37-39] Treatment approaches appropriate for postural education may include neuro-developmental treatment,[40] proprioceptive neuromuscular facilitation,[41] and Feldenkrais techniques.[42]

Specific exercises for encouraging development of motor mile-

FIGURE 15. Five-month-old infant with right torticollis working on weight shifting and reaching in prone by (a) reaching to the right, (b) reaching to the left. Infant has greater difficulty righting her head and shifting weight to reach to the uninvolved side.

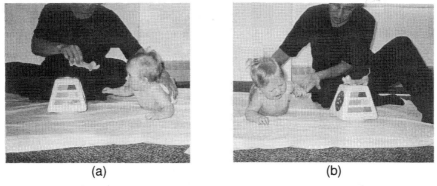

(a)   (b)

FIGURE 16. Same 5-month-old infant with right torticollis working on neck and trunk strengthening in (a) sidelying on right, (b) sidelying on left, (c) prone reaching left, (d) prone reaching right.

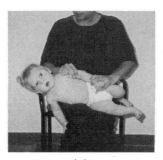   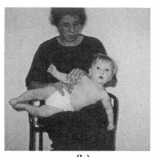

(a)   (b)

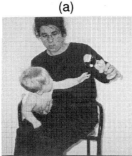   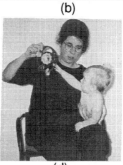

(c)   (d)

FIGURE 17. Same 5-month-old infant with right torticollis working on active neck and trunk rotation to the right in sitting.

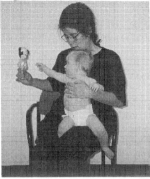

FIGURE 18. Four-year-old child with left torticollis working on right side asymmetrical neck extension strengthening in prone.

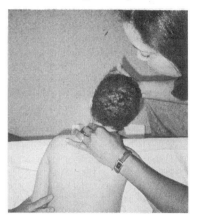

stones are added if the patient displays any developmental asymmetry or delay in motor skill function. Areas in which we commonly observe delay are: prone skills, symmetry in weight shifts and weight-bearing, midline control, upper extremity midline activity, and symmetry in transitional movement skills.

Frequency and Duration of Treatment

Frequency of visits will depend on the level of involvement, age of the child, and parents' ability to perform a home-based program successfully. Initially, the patient can be seen twice a week, weekly, or bi-monthly. Visits are spaced out as adequate ROM and strength is achieved, parents become confident with home-based exercise, and the patient demonstrates acquisition of functional control of head positioning combined with dynamic play in all areas of motor skill development. Emery has used regression analysis to model treatment duration based on severity of SCM muscle involvement at entry to treatment.[23] Average duration for complete recovery of full passive neck range of motion was 4.7 months.[23]

Anticipated Outcomes

A child may achieve (1) full passive symmetrical ROM of neck and trunk; (2) active symmetrical head rotation from a midline position to 80° left and right in prone, supine, sit and stand; (3) active midline head to trunk alignment during static and dynamic play with intermittent head tilt toward the involved side; (4) good antigravity trunk and neck strength with symmetry between uninvolved and involved sides; (5) symmetry between left and right sides in righting and equilibrium reactions in both the horizontal and vertical planes; and (6) ability to assume head tilt toward the uninvolved side with or without rotation to the involved side during play activities involving either static or dynamic postures. These anticipated outcomes of intervention are listed from easiest to achieve to more difficult. Parents often continue to work on strength and postural education after the therapist has discharged the child from intervention. Full active and passive ROM of the neck and trunk should be achieved prior to discharge, and it is most important to educate the family in a home-based program.

In summary, a good history and clinical examination will exclude many conditions which may cause a torticollis posture.[43,44] Differential diagnosis should exclude ocular causes and musculoskeletal anomalies. A radiological examination of the cervical spine may be necessary before manual therapy is begun. A therapy program should emphasize neck and trunk strengthening and mobility, midline postural control, symmetry of postural responses, symmetry of weight-bearing and transitional movements, and age-appropriate motor skill development.

REFERENCES

1. Jones PG. *Torticollis in Infancy and Childhood.* Springfield, IL: Charles C Thomas; 1968.

2. Binder H, Eng GD, Gaiser JF et al. Congenital muscular torticollis: results of conservative management with long-term follow-up in 85 cases. *Arch Phys Med Rehabil.* 1987; 68:222-225.

3. Shapiro IJ. Relationship between vertical facial asymmetry and postural changes of the spine and ancillary muscles. *Optometry and Vision Science.* 1994; 71(8):529-538.

4. Wolfort FG, Kanter MA, Miller LB. Torticollis. *Plastic and Reconstructive Surgery.* 1989; 84:682-692.

5. Morrison DL, MacEwen GD. Congenital muscular torticollis: observations regarding clinical finds, associated conditions, and results of treatment. *J Pediatr Orthop.* 1982; 2:500-505.

6. Kendall FP, McCreary EK, Provance PG. *Muscles Testing and Function,* 4th Ed. Baltimore, MD: Williams & Wilkins; 1993.

7. Ling CM, Low YS. Sternomastoid tumor and muscular torticollis. *Clin Orthopaed Rel Research.* 1972; 86:144-150.

8. MacDonald D. Sternomastoid tumor and muscular torticollis. *J Bone Joint Surg.* 1969; 51(B):432.

9. Anderson W. Clinical lecture on sternomastoid torticollis. *Lancet.* 1893; 1:9.

10. Ruedmann AD. Scoliosis and vertical ocular muscle imbalance. *Arch Ophthalmol.* 1956; 56:389-414.

11. Kapandji IA. *The Physiology of the Joints. Vol 3. The Trunk and Vertebral Column,* 2nd ed. London, UK: Churchill Livingstone; 1974.

12. Upledger JR, Vredevoogd JD. *Craniosacral Therapy.* Seattle, WA: Eastland Press; 1983.

13. Ferte AD. The role of the platysma muscle in torticollis deformity. *Plastic Reconstructive Surgery.* 1947; 2:72.

14. Caputo AR, Mickey KJ, Guo S et al. The sit-up test: an alternate clinical test for evaluating pediatric torticollis. *Pediatrics.* 1992; 90:612-614.

15. Rubin ER, Wagner RS. Occular torticollis. *Survey of Ophthalmology.* 1986; 30:366-376.

16. Bruno B, Emilio CC, Carlo C. Plagiocephaly causing superior oblique deficiency and occular torticollis. *Archives Ophthalmology.* 1982; 100:1093-1096.

17. Vander Kolk CA, Carson BS. Lambdoid synostosis. *Craniofacial Surgery.* 1994; 21:575-584.

18. Coventry MB, Harris LE. Congenital muscular torticollis in infancy. *J Bone Joint Surg.* 1959; 41(A):815.

19. Poole MD, Griggs M. The cranio-facio-cervical scoliosis complex. *Br J Plastic Surg.* 1990; 43:670-675.

20. Putnam GD, Postlethwaite KR, Chate RA et al. Facial scoliosis—a diagnostic dilemma. *Int J Oral Maxillofac Surg.* 1993; 22:324-327.

21. Ferkel RD, Westin GW, Dawson EG. Muscular torticollis. *J Bone Joint Surg.* 1983; 65(7):894-900.

22. Cloni G, Prechtl HFR. Pre-term and early post-term motor behavior in low-risk premature infants. *Early Human Development.* 1990; 23:159-191.

23. Emery C. The determinants of treatment duration for congenital muscular torticollis. *Phys Ther.* 1994; 74:921-929.

24. Youdas JW, Carey JR, Garrett TR. Reliability of measurements of cervical spine range of motion-comparison of three methods. *Phys Ther.* 1991; 71:98-106.

25. Campbell SK, Kolobe THA, Osten ET et al. Construct validity of the Test of Infant Motor Performance. *Phys Ther.* 1995; 75:585-596.

26. Ellison PH, Horn JL, Browning CA. Construction of an Infant Neurological International Battery (INFANIB) for the assessment of neurological integrity in infancy. *Phys Ther.* 1985; 65:1326-1331.

27. King-Thomas L, Hacker BJ. *A Therapist's Guide to Pediatric Assessment.* Boston, MA: Little, Brown, and Company; 1987: 185-189.

28. Chandler LS, Andrews MS, Swanson MW. *Movement Assessment of Infants: A Manual.* Rolling Bay, WA; 1980.

29. Bayley N. *Bayley II.* San Antonio, TX: Psychological Corporation; 1994.

30. Andre-Thomas, Chesni Y, Dargassies SS. *The Neurological Examination of the Infant.* London, UK: National Spastics Society; 1960:11-50.

31. Connolly BH, Montgomery PC. *Therapeutic Exercise in Developmental Disabilities.* Chattanooga, TN: Chattanooga Corporation; 1987: 55-73.

32. Mazzini L, Schieppati M. Short-latency neck muscle responses to vertical body tilt in normal subjects and in patients with spasmodic torticollis. *Electroencephalogr Clin Neurophysiol.* 1994; 93:265-275.

33. Dutia MB. The muscles and joints of the neck: their specialisation and role in head movement. *Prog Neurobiol.* 1991; 37:165-178.

34. Davids JR, Wenger OR, Mubarak SH. Congenital muscular torticollis: sequela of intrauterine or perinatal component syndrome. *Journal of Pediatric Orthopaedics.* 1993; 13:141-147.

35. Mirabelli L, Pain management. In: Umphred DA, ed. *Neurological Rehabilitation.* St. Louis, Mo: CV Mosby Company; 1985: 600-615.

36. Wilbarger P. Planning an adequate sensory diet, application of sensory processing theory during the first year of life. *Zero to Three.* September, 1994: 7-12.

37. Shumway-Cook A, Woollacott M. The growth of stability: postural control from a developmental perspective. *J Motor Behavior.* 1985; 17:131-147.

38. Shumway-Cook A, Woollacott M. Theoretical issues in assessing postural control. In: Wilhelm IJ, ed. *Physical Therapy Assessment in Early Infancy.* New York, NY: Churchill Livingstone; 1993:161-171.

39. Campbell SK. The child's development of functional movement. In: Campbell SK, Vander Linden DW, Palisano RJ. *Physical Therapy for Children.* Philadelphia, PA: WB Saunders; 1994:3-37.

40. Girolami GL, Campbell SK. Efficacy of a Neuro-developmental Treatment Program to Improve Motor Control in Infants Born Prematurely. *Pediatric Physical Therapy;* 1994, 6:175-184.

41. Sullivan PE, Markos PD, Minor MA. *An Integrated Approach to Therapeutic Exercise*. Reston, VA: Reston Publishing Company; 1982.

42. Feldenkrais M. *Awareness Through Movement*. New York, NY: Harper and Row Publishers; 1977.

43. Brendenkamp JK, Maceri DP. Inflammatory torticollis in children. *Arch Otolaryngol Head Neck Surg*. 1990; 116:310-313.

44. Tom LWC, Rossiter JR et al. Torticollis in children. *Otolaryngol Head Neck Surg*. 1991; 105:1-5.

The Surgical Management
of Congenital Muscular Torticollis

Ashwani Rajput
Michael W. L. Gauderer

SUMMARY. The majority of children with congenital muscular torticollis are successfully treated with an aggressive physical therapy program. A select group of patients, however, clearly require an operation for a successful outcome. This article takes a historical look at the role of surgery in the management of congenital muscular torticollis and its evolution into today's management principles. By reviewing the literature, we define the subset of children requiring an operation and the ideal timing of the operation. Finally, a brief description of the operative intervention is given. *[Article copies available for a fee from The Haworth Document Delivery Service: 1-800-342-9678. E-mail address: getinfo@haworth.com]*

HISTORY

The occurrence of congenital muscular torticollis (CMT) has been documented in many ancient writings.[1] In fact, it is speculated

---

Ashwani Rajput, MD, is Resident Physician, Dudley P. Allen Research Scholar, and Clinical Instructor, Department of Surgery, Case Western Reserve University, Cleveland, OH. Michael W. L. Gauderer is Chief, Department of Pediatric Surgery, The Children's Hospital, Greenville Hospital System, Greenville, SC.

Address correspondence to: Michael W. L. Gauderer, MD, Memorial Medical Office Building, 890 West Faris Road, Suite 440, Greenville, SC 29605.

[Haworth co-indexing entry note]: "The Surgical Management of Congenital Muscular Torticollis." Rajput, Ashwani, and Michael W. L. Gauderer. Co-published simultaneously in *Physical & Occupational Therapy in Pediatrics* (The Haworth Press, Inc.) Vol. 17, No. 2, 1997, pp. 69-80; and: *Torticollis: Differential Diagnosis, Assessment and Treatment, Surgical Management and Bracing* (ed: Karen Karmel-Ross) The Haworth Press, Inc., 1997, pp. 69-80. Single or multiple copies of this article are available for a fee from The Haworth Document Delivery Service [1-800-342-9678, 9:00 a.m. - 5:00 p.m. (EST). E-mail address: getinfo@haworth.com].

that Alexander the Great suffered from muscular torticollis because he had a "lifting of the neck with a slight bending to the left."[2]

The history of the surgical management of muscular torticollis is not documented quite as far back as the time of Alexander the Great (356-323 BC), but it is still an ancient and colorful story. Antyllus (c350 AD) is credited with performing the first tenotomy for a joint contracture, but it is not known whether he ever operated on the sternocleidomastoid (SCM) muscle.[1] The first documentation of tenotomy for torticollis is provided by a friend and the personal physician of Rembrandt, Nicholaes Tulp (1593-1694). In his book *Observationes Medicae*, Tulp described a child with a wry neck since birth who at the age of twelve years underwent a tenotomy.[3] The operation was performed by Isacius Minnius who was recommended because of previous successful operations.

Around the same time period, certain less reputable individuals in England were performing a similar operation. The vicar of Stratford-on-Avon (1663-1681), John Ward, documents the activities at the *fairgrounds* as follows:

> . . . the mountebank that cuts wry necks, cutt three tendons in one child's neck, and hee did it thus. First by making a small orifice with his Launcett and lifting upp the tendons for fear of the jugular veins, and cutting them upwards; they give a great snap when cutt. The orifice of his wounds are small and scarce any blood follows.[4(p 9)]

During the eighteenth century, the operative treatment of muscular torticollis fell into disrepute. Although not commonly performed, it was recorded in the English medical literature by Sharp in 1740.[5] He described the division of the sternomastoid muscle at the junction of its middle and lower thirds. The space between the muscles was plugged with lint to prevent early reunion. By the nineteenth century, the sternomastoid tenotomy was rediscovered by Baron Dupuytren, a surgeon in Napoleonic France. He wrote:

> . . . he always made a puncture in the skin near the medial border of the lower end of the sternomastoid, through which he introduced the flat side of blunt-ended bistoury along the deep surface of the muscle, as far as the outer border of the cleidomastoid tendon: then turning the cutting edge of the

instrument towards the muscle, he severed it from behind forwards without cutting the skin.[6(p 10)]

As the surgical treatment for torticollis evolved, Mikulicz in 1895 recommended the complete excision of the sternomastoid muscle which contained the tumor.[7] To evaluate the necessity for complete excision, Pollard in 1896 followed 23 infants with a sternomastoid tumor. He found that in the majority of infants, the muscle returned to normal during the first year of life.[8] Thus, there was no evidence for the total excision of the muscle in all children diagnosed with a sternomastoid mass as proposed by Mikulicz.[7]

Surgeons at the end of the twentieth century agree with Pollard's observations at the end of the nineteenth century. In fact, up to 80% of patients with a mass in the (SCM) respond to conservative therapy (i.e., positioning, exercise, and massage).[9,10] The other 20% of patients will require division of the affected SCM; therefore, it is important for the clinician to determine which children require an operative intervention (Figures 1 and 2).

FIGURE 1. Typical torticollis in a two-month-old girl. Although the right SCM mass is fairly large, the lesion resolved fully with physical therapy only. This is the usual course.

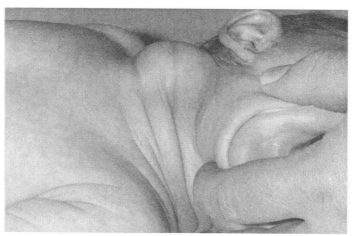

FIGURE 2. Four-month-old boy with severe right torticollis not responsive to intense physical therapy. Head deformity with skull asymmetry was already apparent. The mother and two of her siblings also had torticollis, eventually requiring transection of the muscle.

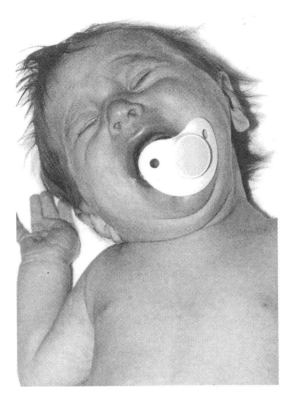

GOALS AND TIMING OF OPERATION

The main goals of treatment are for improving: (1) neck range-of-motion, (2) cosmesis, and (3) function. For those patients not responding to conservative therapy, the surgeon must decide when the appropriate time is to operate so that the above stated goals may be met.

To help provide guidelines for the timing of treatment, Canale and associates reviewed their experience with 57 patients with

CMT.[11] Of the original 57 patients, 28 required surgical release. The average follow-up period was 18.9 years. Upon follow-up, cosmetic and functional results were documented. A cosmetic result was deemed satisfactory if the patient had no facial asymmetry, no head tilt, and no palpable tightness of the SCM muscle. An unsatisfactory cosmetic result was documented if facial asymmetry was present, and there was a residual contracture of the SCM muscle, with or without head tilt. Functional results were considered satisfactory if the patient had full rotation of the head or loss of rotation of less than 30 degrees. An unsatisfactory functional result was documented when the patient had a loss of rotation of 30 degrees or more, with or without discomfort.

The results of functional and cosmetic outcomes were combined, and patients were scored as having a good, fair, or poor outcome. The definitions of the scoring system is as follows:

Good: satisfactory functional AND cosmetic outcome
Fair: unsatisfactory functional OR cosmetic outcome
Poor: unsatisfactory functional AND cosmetic outcome

Overall outcomes were also analyzed based on patient age at the time treatment was initiated. Group I consisted of patients treated before the age of one year; Group II included patients treated between the ages of 1 and 10 years; and Group III was comprised of those treated after the age of 10 years.

Upon analyzing their data, the authors concluded that children who are treated in the first year of life have better results then those treated later regardless of the type of treatment.[11] Non-operative therapy, however, was likely to be unsuccessful if the restriction of rotation was more than 30 degrees, if significant facial asymmetry was present, and if the child was older than 1 year.

Morrison and MacEwen reviewed 232 patients with CMT and also attempted to answer the question as to the ideal timing of repair.[12] They concluded that "there appears to be no justification for a surgical approach in the child with congenital muscular torticollis under 1 year of age."[12(p 500)]

In another study, Ippolito and associates evaluated the results of open SCM tenotomy in 67 patients with CMT and identified factors that most affected the outcome of surgical treatment.[13] The patients were divided into 3 groups depending on their age at the time of operation. The groups were defined as follows:

Group I: operation between the ages of 5 months and 6 years
Group II: operation between the ages of 7 and 11 years
Group III: operation at 12 years or older

The outcomes were rated by the system developed by Canale and colleagues[11] as defined above as good, fair, and poor. Thirty-seven percent of the patients had a good result, 45% had a fair, and 18% had a poor result. Those patients in Group I had the best results and those in Group III the worst. Based on their data, the authors concluded that, in general, the patient's age at operation, the duration of the condition and the severity of the deformity before the operation had the major effects on both cosmetic and functional results.

Largely based on the above referenced work, it is generally agreed that surgical intervention for the treatment of CMT should not be undertaken in patients less than one year of age. As previously cited, 80% of patients may have a resolution of the condition with non-operative means and achieve a good result. Neither a decrease in the range of motion, nor the development of plagiocephaly should alone dictate an operation because improvement in both conditions can occur. If, however, facial hemihypoplasia is diagnosed, the patient should be considered for an operation regardless of age. There has been no documentation that facial hemihypoplasia regresses without operation once it has begun to develop.[1]

THE OPERATION

The patient is placed in the supine position on the operating table with the head turned slightly toward the direction opposite the involved muscle. An incision is made in one of the tension lines of the skin. This is simple and has a good cosmetic result (Figures 3-7). The muscle is dissected at the level where the sternal and clavicular heads converge. The central portion of the muscle is removed. Additional tissue is excised as needed because the amount of fibrosis of the fascia varies from case to case. Usually, the fascia colli is incised from the anterior border of the trapezius muscle to the anterior midline. In cases of severe torticollis, the fascia around

FIGURE 3. Pre-operative view with the SCM muscle maximally stretched. Notice the broad, flat appearance.

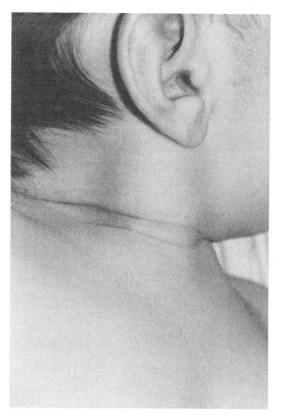

the carotid sheath and omohyoid muscle are also released.[14] Prior to closure, the head is fully rotated while a finger palpates the wound to find any residual bands requiring division. The wound is then closed, without drainage, with a running subcuticular suture.

A dry dressing is placed over the wound. A soft bulky pad is added and the neck is wrapped loosely with cotton gauze. Slight neck hyperextension is desirable (Figure 5). Physical therapy is resumed one to two weeks following the operation depending on the patient's tolerance (see Jacques and Karmel-Ross, this volume, for information on post-operative bracing treatment).

FIGURE 4. Operative photograph. Hemostat elevating the SCM muscle. Notice the intensely white, tendon-like appearance of the muscle. The resected specimen was composed primarily of fibrous tissue.

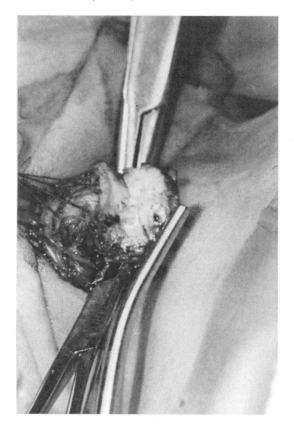

CONCLUSION

As with many disease processes in medicine, CMT has a spectrum in its presentation. Some patients are mildly affected, whereas others are severely impaired. The majority of patients respond to aggressive conservative therapy. Surgery, however, clearly has a role in a select population of patients with CMT. This population mainly consists of those individuals who have not responded to

FIGURE 5. Postoperative splinting, hyperextending the neck.

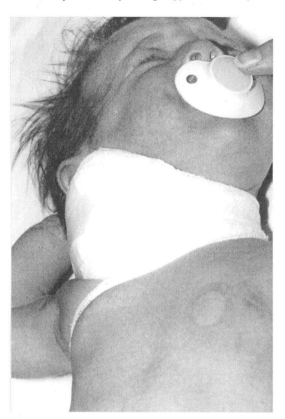

conservative therapy by the age of one year or any child displaying facial hemihypoplasia regardless of age.

Once the diagnosis of CMT is made, it is important to have a surgeon involved in the care of the patient. In severe cases, the surgeon should see the patient at least once a month to assess the progress of physical therapy. As soon as hemihypoplasia is seen, physical therapy should be intensified and an operative plan should be considered.

The surgeon, however, is not the only person involved in achieving a good outcome in a child with CMT. The importance of a team approach to management cannot be overstated. Parents and primary

FIGURE 6. Follow-up photograph four months later. Four years later the child is normal with a full range of motion. This is the youngest patient on whom we performed a transection of the SCM muscle.

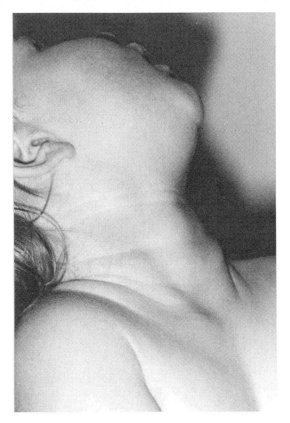

care physicians need to be aware of the condition to achieve early diagnosis. Physical therapists and occupational therapists need to be involved early to set up an effective therapy program. Furthermore, if an operation is needed, a post-operative therapy program is important for a successful outcome. Thus, with a multi-disciplinary approach, health care workers may individualize a treatment approach for each patient and successfully meet the goals of achieving function and cosmesis in caring for a child with CMT (Figures 6 and 7).

FIGURE 7. Three-year-old boy, two years after transection of left SCM muscle. Although the muscle is virtually absent, he has normal range of motion.

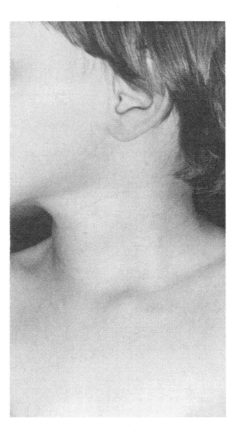

REFERENCES

1. Jones P. *Torticollis in Infancy and Childhood.* Springfield, IL: Charles C Thomas; 1968.

2. Plutarch, in Jones P. *Torticollis in Infancy and Childhood.* Springfield, IL: Charles C Thomas; 1968: 3.

3. Tulp N, in Jones P. *Torticollis in Infancy and Childhood.* Springfield, IL: Charles C Thomas; 1968: 7.

4. Power, in Jones P. *Torticollis in Infancy and Childhood.* Springfield, IL: Charles C Thomas; 1968: 9.

5. Sharp, in Jones P. *Torticollis in Infancy and Childhood.* Springfield, IL: Charles C Thomas; 1968: 10.

6. Dupuytren, in Jones P. *Torticollis in Infancy and Childhood.* Springfield, IL: Charles C Thomas; 1968:10-11.

7. Mikulicz, in Jones P. *Torticollis in Infancy and Childhood.* Springfield, IL: Charles C Thomas; 1968: 13.

8. Pollard, in Jones P. *Torticollis in Infancy and Childhood.* Springfield, IL: Charles C Thomas; 1968: 13.

9. Grosfeld J. Pediatric Surgery. In: Sabiston D, ed. *Textbook of Surgery: The Biologic Basis of Modern Surgical Practice.* Philadelphia, PA: WB Saunders Company; 1991:1177.

10. Binder H, Eng GD, Gaiser JF et al. Congenital muscular torticollis: results of conservative management with long-term follow-up in 85 cases. *Arch Phys Med Rehabil.* 1985; 68:222-225.

11. Canale ST, Griffin DW, Hubbard CN. Congenital muscular torticollis. *J Bone and Joint Surg.* 1982; 64:810-816.

12. Morrison DL, MacEwen GD. Congenital muscular torticollis: observations regarding clinical findings, associated conditions and results of treatment. *J Pediatr Orthop.* 1982;2:500-505.

13. Ippolito E, Tudisco D, Massobiro M. Long-term results of open sternocleidomastoid tenotomy for idiopathic muscular torticollis. *J Bone and Joint Surg.* 1985;67:30-38.

14. Jones PG. Torticollis. In Welch KJ, Randolph JG, Ravitch MM et al., eds. *Pediatric Surgery.* Chicago. Year Book Medical Publishers, Inc; 1986:552-556.

The Use of Splinting in Conservative and Post-Operative Treatment of Congenital Muscular Torticollis

Carole Jacques
Karen Karmel-Ross

SUMMARY. Standard conservative treatment for infants with congenital muscular torticollis does not consistently resolve lateral head tilt. This paper describes two custom-made neck collars used for this purpose. Indications for use and fabrication, as well as precautions, are discussed. Collars are readily accepted as part of the treatment program and are effective in improving the infant's ability to hold his or her head in midline. In addition, a procedure for splinting following surgery to lengthen the sternocleidomastoid muscle is described. *[Article copies available for a fee from The Haworth Document Delivery Service: 1-800-342-9678. E-mail address: getinfo@haworth.com]*

Standard conservative treatment[1,2] of infants with congenital muscular torticollis (CMT) consisting of stretching, positioning,

Carole Jacques, BSR, Reg OT(BC), is Clinical Coordinator, Occupational Therapy Department, British Columbia's Children's Hospital, Vancouver, BC, Canada. Karen Karmel-Ross, PT, PCS, LMT, is Pediatric Clinical Specialist, Department of Rehabilitation Services, University Hospitals of Cleveland, Cleveland, OH.

Address correspondence to: Carole Jacques, Occupational Therapy Department, British Columbia's Children's Hospital, 4480 Oak Street, Vancouver, BC V6H 3V4, Canada.

The authors would like to thank Carol Adam Mahony for the illustrations.

[Haworth co-indexing entry note]: "The Use of Splinting in Conservative and Post-Operative Treatment of Congenital Muscular Torticollis." Jacques, Carole, and Karen Karmel-Ross. Co-published simultaneously in *Physical & Occupational Therapy in Pediatrics* (The Haworth Press, Inc.) Vol. 17, No. 2, 1997, pp. 81-90; and: *Torticollis: Differential Diagnosis, Assessment and Treatment, Surgical Management and Bracing* (ed: Karen Karmel-Ross) The Haworth Press, Inc., 1997, pp. 81-90. Single or multiple copies of this article are available for a fee from The Haworth Document Delivery Service [1-800-342-9678, 9:00 a.m. - 5:00 p.m. (EST). E-mail address: getinfo@haworth.com].

and strengthening has been practiced widely throughout North America for the past twenty years. Published results of treatment have been inconsistent in use of assessments and descriptors, making outcomes difficult to analyze. In our clinical experience we have found that full neck range of motion (ROM) was generally achieved within a few months of beginning treatment for infants under one year of age. Some infants, however, continued to show a persistent head tilt toward the side of the torticollis. This led us to develop two types of collar, the Tubular Orthosis for Torticollis (TOT) and a foam collar, to be used as adjuncts in the management of this group of children.

DESCRIPTION

The Tubular Orthosis for Torticollis or TOT[3] is assembled from premade plastic parts; the foam collar is adapted from a small adult-sized cervical collar. Both devices employ a lateral obstruction to limit head tilt toward the side of the torticollis but permit freedom of movement in other directions. We believe that the TOT is somewhat more dynamic than the foam collar; it produces mild discomfort on lateral head tilt, thereby stimulating active lifting of the head away from the noxious input and toward vertical alignment.

INDICATIONS

Collar use is added to the conservative treatment of infants with CMT if they are 4 months of age or older and show a consistent head tilt of 5 degrees or more. The infant must have adequate ROM and lateral head righting reactions (head control and strength) to lift his or her head away from the side of the collar.

FABRICATION AND FIT

Tubular Orthosis for Torticollis*

A length of PVC tubing twice the circumference of the neck plus 4-6 inches is cut and joined into a circle using an end connector

---

*TOT collar available in Canada from Symmetric Designs Ltd, Ganges, BC, (604) 537-2177, and in the U.S. from North Coast Medical, San Jose, CA, 1-800-821-9319.

(Figure 1). Two struts to provide a lateral stimulus on the affected side are selected, allowing .5 inch for T-junctions at the top and bottom: strut A spans from posterior to the crest of the trapezius to the occiput and strut B from anterior to the crest of the trapezius to the tip of the mastoid process. A T-junction is fitted over the PVC tubing approximately 1 inch from the end connector and inserted into strut A. A second T-junction is similarly positioned on the other side of the end connector and inserted into the other end of strut A. Strut B is joined to the PVC tubing about 1 inch from strut A at one end and about 3 inches away at the other end, using two more T-junctions (Figure 2). The ends of the collar are fastened together with a C-clip. Occasionally, the end connector can cause skin irritation and pressure when placed centrally. An alternative in this case is to place the end connector along the base of the neck and join the PVC tubing by tying it at the side of the neck with twill tape (Figure 3).

The collar is placed on the infant and any necessary adjustments are made to length and position of struts and length of PVC tubing. For correct fit, the infant should be holding his or her head in midline, slightly away from the struts, and there should be room for 1 or 2 adult-sized fingers to fit between the C-clip and the back of the neck, or between the PVC tubing and the anterior neck.

To increase comfort and decrease the likelihood of pinching the skin, moleskin can be wrapped around the two layers of PVC tubing in the area under the chin. The struts and T-junctions can also be covered with moleskin although this makes it more difficult to

FIGURE 1. TOT Parts: A, End Connector; B, T-Junction; C, C-Clip; D, Strut

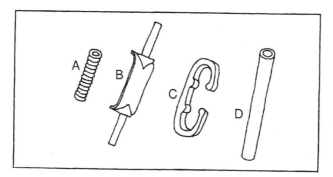

FIGURE 2. Completed Collar

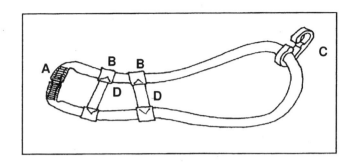

FIGURE 3. Alternative Method of Fastening TOT

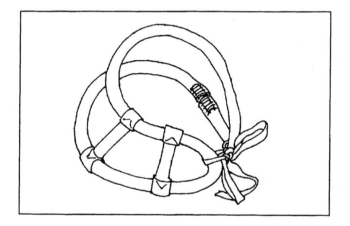

adjust the fit of the collar. Alternatively, the collar can be placed inside a sleeve of stockinette.

Foam Collar

Choose an adult-sized small, firm foam cervical collar with adequate length to fit around the infant's neck. Remove the stockinette and velcro to expose the foam. Cut the foam to be narrow under the chin and on the uninvolved side. A concave section may be cut out under the ear on the involved side to avoid pressure to the ear lobe. The collar will attach at the middle of the back of the neck. The collar on the involved side should support the head as close to midline as possible. Decreasing the height and thinning the foam on the uninvolved side and under the chin will allow the child to laterally flex toward that side. The collar should be as vertical as possible. There should be room for 1 or 2 adult-sized fingers to fit between the neck and collar. A good place to check this is in the front of the neck during swallowing. The collar is covered with cotton fabric and velcro closures are sewn on (Figure 4).

APPLICATION AND USE

Application of the collar is generally easiest with the young infant in prone. The center of the TOT is placed under the chin, the struts positioned spanning the shoulder on the affected side, with the top of the anterior strut on the mastoid process (just behind the earlobe). The C-clip is then fastened (Figure 5). The foam collar is positioned similarly, with the highest aspect under the ear on the affected side (Figure 6). As both infant and caregiver become more accustomed to the process, the collar can be put on with the infant sitting or standing.

Because the TOT is easily adjusted, it can initially be made to fit

FIGURE 4. Foam Collar

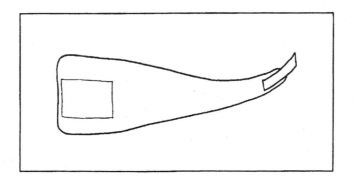

FIGURE 5. Child Wearing TOT

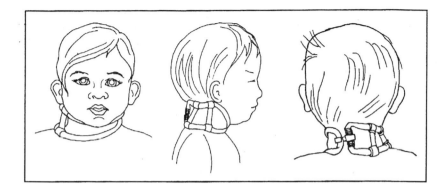

FIGURE 6. Child Wearing Foam Collar

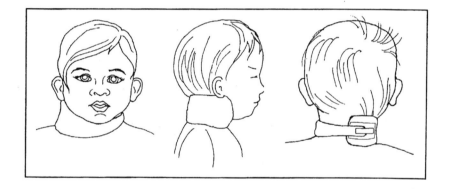

looser than is optimal in order to facilitate the build-up of wearing tolerance and the learning of application by caregivers. The goal is full-time wear during the waking hours and most infants achieve this within the first week (toddlers may require a bit longer). TOT fit is then adjusted by changing the length of struts or tubing to stimulate active correction of head position to achieve midline orientation. Further adjustments are made as required for growth. The collar is removed for stretches. Active strengthening exercises may be done while wearing the collar. We find that collar wear is generally required for a minimum of 2 to 3 months and may be needed for 8 months or more in some instances.

The infant's head position without the collar is reassessed at each clinic visit. When head tilt is less than 5 degrees consistently, collar use is gradually decreased. The collar is removed for 1 to 2 hours at a time of day when the infant is most rested and likely to maintain a good head position (often on rising in the morning or following naps). Head position is monitored by the parent at these times. If a midline position is maintained consistently, time without wearing the collar is gradually extended. The collar is reapplied if head tilt recurs. This may be seen near nap times, at the end of the day, or following exercise sessions when the muscles are fatigued. Head tilt may also increase with teething or when the child is ill.

PRECAUTIONS

Collar use is intended to stimulate muscle activation for correction of head position to midline orientation. If the infant is unable to achieve this position, he may use the collar as a passive support or may adjust his body position to avoid correction. The therapist must watch for depression of the shoulder on the affected side, trunk curvature, or lateral shifting of the cervical spine. All infants should have visual screening to eliminate the possibility of visual torticollis before applying a collar.

Some children are reluctant to turn their head toward the affected side while wearing the collar because it does provide some resistance to this movement. Extra emphasis should be placed on gaining neck rotation toward the affected side both in the clinic and at home.

Caution must be taken when applying the collar to avoid pinching or folding the skin under the tubing or edge of the foam. Infants often show considerable redness under the TOT tubing and struts after a period of wear. Parents must be instructed in checking the skin periodically after removal of the collar. Redness should fade within a half-hour.

During hot weather some children may develop a heat rash while wearing a collar. Use of talcum powder or corn starch helps to keep the skin dry. The TOT can be enclosed in a sleeve of stockinette or other soft fabric to improve comfort.

OUTCOME

Our clinical observation of infants with CMT demonstrated that, although conservative treatment of CMT improved muscle length and strength, some infants and children did not adopt an upright head position. We believe that the addition to the treatment program of the use of a custom-made collar which stimulates active use of the contralateral sternocleidomastoid (SCM) muscle throughout the day results in improved strength of that muscle and a more consistently upright position of the head. Infants who also have plagiocephaly may have improved symmetry if collar use is initiated early.

A small pilot study on the use of the TOT was conducted at British Columbia's Children's Hospital (BCCH) in 1984-85.[3] The group of infants fitted with a TOT had an average head position of 89.5 degrees (90 degrees = vertical) at the end of treatment; the control group had an average head position of 84.8 degrees.

The use of a collar as an adjunct to conservative treatment of CMT has been readily accepted by parents, children, and infants, and we have noted no deleterious effects. Its use with infants with CMT over 4 months of age who consistently have a head tilt of more than 5 degrees has become a routine part of our management program for these infants.

POST-SURGICAL SPLINTING FOR CMT

At BCCH, orthopaedic surgeons see several new patients each year with untreated or unresolved CMT. Following surgical lengthening or release of the SCM, the surgeons prefer to have the child's head maintained in a position that prevents re-shortening of the muscle during healing. To achieve the desired positioning, occupational therapists enter the operating room immediately following the surgical procedure to fabricate a low temperature thermoplastic "collar" while the child remains under anaesthetic. Over the years this collar has taken numerous forms; the present version is a hybrid of a design developed at BCCH with one from Sick Children's Hospital in Toronto, Ontario, Canada.

The child's head is positioned such that the previously shortened muscle is placed on stretch–that is, tilted laterally away from the released muscle and rotated toward it. Jobst custom-splint thermoplastic material (Remington Medical, 1124 Lonsdale Avenue, #406, North Vancouver, B.C., Canada V7M 2H1, phone 1-800-267-5822) is used with contour foam placed for comfort over the jawline, the shoulder on the side opposite the surgery, and any bony prominences, such as the clavicles. Contour foam is also placed over the ear on the surgical side. The premeasured and pre-cut thermoplastic material is molded over the surgical side of the face and skull, the entire neck and both shoulders (Figure 7).

A rolled reinforcement bar of thermoplastic is added to the surgical side to strengthen the splint. The foam is replaced in the jaw and shoulder areas and covered with moleskin. The impression from the foam over the ear is perforated to facilitate hearing. Straps are added to hold the splint down onto the chest and shoulders and to keep it firmly in contact with the skull. The splint is worn 23 hours a day (off for skin care, stretching and exercises) for the first 1 to 2 post-surgical months and at night for several more months. We believe that use of this splint has been effective in maintaining length of the SCM muscle following surgery.

FIGURE 7. Child Wearing Post-Surgical Splint

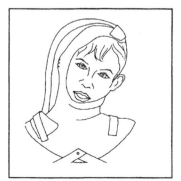

CONCLUSION

Two custom-fabricated collars for use as adjuncts to conservative treatment of CMT and an orthosis for post-surgical maintenance of lengthening of the SCM muscle were described. Orthotic aids are believed to be useful for improving vertical alignment of the head on the trunk in management of congenital muscular torticollis.

REFERENCES

1. Fabian K, Marshall M. Conservative and surgical treatment of congenital muscular torticollis: a literature review. *Physiother Canada.* 1984; 36:146-151.

2. Binder H, Eng G, Gaiser JF et al. Congenital muscular torticollis: results of conservative management with long term follow-up in 85 cases. *Arch Phys Med Rehabil.* 1987; 68:222-225.

3. Cottrill-Mosterman S, Jacques C, Bartlett D et al. Orthotic treatment of head tilt in children with congenital muscular torticollis. *J Assoc Children's Prosthetic-Orthotic Clinics.* 1987; 22(1-3).

Infants with Torticollis:
The Relationship Between Asymmetric Head and Neck Positioning and Postural Development

Nancy Hylton

SUMMARY. This article explores the effect of perinatal injury of the sternocleidomastoid muscle on general postural and movement development in the first year of life. The focus is on infants with no obvious generalized movement problems and no observable on-going muscle pathology. Residual, strong torticollis retained past four months of age appears to have a profound effect on internal sensory maps or body image formation, as well as on the midline axial postural stability and patterns of surface loading necessary for move-

Nancy Hylton, PT, is Pediatric Therapist, Consultant and Co-Founder, Children's Therapy Center of Kent, Kent, WA.

Address correspondence to: Nancy Hylton, Children's Therapy Center of Kent, 10811 Kent-Kangley Road, Kent, WA 98031.

The author would like to express her deepest appreciation to Berta Bobath and Mary Quinton for foundational understandings of postural control and movement and a creative, ever expanding approach to therapy. Appreciation also goes to Dr. Karl Bobath and Dr. Elizabeth Köng for instilling the persistent need to try to answer the question "Why?" Very special thanks to all the staff and families of CTC of Kent who enable creative treatment approaches to flourish, to Felicia and her family for continuing to teach the author, and to Shelby Clayson, MS, PT, for the exciting pieces of neural research she shared in a recent course. Special thanks also to Suzann Campbell for superb editing of the author's sometimes convoluted language into understandable form.

[Haworth co-indexing entry note]: "Infants with Torticollis: The Relationship Between Asymmetric Head and Neck Positioning and Postural Development." Hylton, Nancy. Co-published simultaneously in *Physical & Occupational Therapy in Pediatrics* (The Haworth Press, Inc.) Vol. 17, No. 2, 1997, pp. 91-117; and: *Torticollis: Differential Diagnosis, Assessment and Treatment, Surgical Management and Bracing* (ed: Karen Karmel-Ross) The Haworth Press, Inc., 1997, pp. 91-117. Single or multiple copies of this article are available for a fee from The Haworth Document Delivery Service [1-800-342-9678, 9:00 a.m. - 5:00 p.m. (EST). E-mail address: getinfo@haworth.com].

ment and balance development. Torticollis also appears to diminish
the infant's ability to organize postural responses, especially ventral
trunk muscle activation in response to backwards displacement. The
article explores these clinical observations and describes one sensorimotor approach to therapeutic intervention for these infants. *[Article
copies available for a fee from The Haworth Document Delivery Service:
1-800-342-9678. E-mail address: getinfo@haworth.com]*

TYPICAL DEVELOPMENT OF POSTURAL CONTROL

Prone Position

Young infants rely upon neck righting responses to manage anti-
gravity movements and generate stabilizing postural connections
with surfaces. The newborn's urge to lift the head in prone and to
turn it from side to side weights the fists, lower rib cage, and knees
in a characteristic manner. This position necessitates forceful upper
back and end-range neck extension to support head movement.[1] By
three to four months of age the characteristic weight bearing pattern
in prone position has become much broader in terms of surface
contact with forearms, abdomen and medial leg contact with the
surface. The posture is associated with extension in upper, middle
and lower spine. The broader base provides greater mechanical
stability from which to activate more complex and differentiated
postural activity. By six to eight months of age, the characteristic
weight bearing contact has again shifted, now to the lateral border
of the hands, lower abdomen, pelvis and anterior thighs. This posture allows a posterior shift of the center of mass, and by producing
a loading into the surface of the lower abdomen, pelvis, and thighs,
frees the arms for reaching activities.[2] Active, graded and balanced
neck extension and stabilization are critical components of each of
these stages of prone postural development. Active chin tuck or
capital flexion is directly related to the amount of dynamic postural
control of the neck and support structures of the body and is
associated with increasing activation of the anterior trunk
muscles.[1-3]

Supine Position

Similarly, in the supine position typical postures combine actively to produce symmetrical head position, chin tuck, and anterior

shoulder, trunk, pelvis and hip muscle activation in association with controlled antigravity arm and leg movements Active head centering in supine develops between 9 and 12 weeks of age and is well established by 15 weeks.[4] As the pattern matures, posterior neck elongation increases, stimulated by visual interest in hands, knees and feet.[1] The period around three to four months of age is characterized by a relatively strong midline orientation, with hands held away from the body high over the chest and touching in midline. Hand movements evoke intense visual interest.[1,5] Activation of the abdominal muscles connects the lower body into this midline orientation, and the feet often touch and play against each other. Body righting responses are temporally associated with the appearance of symmetrical total body postural activation, as seen when active head turning to the side is followed by arms, legs and trunk to reorient the body midline with the midline of the head. A characteristic roll to the sidelying position results. By six to eight months of age, deliberately graded neck rotation is used to recruit and reinforce side-to-side weight-shifting and increasingly refined balance responses in the trunk, limb girdles, arms and legs.[2] Having developed the ability to orient the midline of the head along the midline of the trunk, the infant now organizes postural mechanisms for balance around that central plane.

Refinement of active neck, shoulder, trunk, pelvis and hip postural control requires an increasingly balanced interaction among anterior and posterior, deep and more superficial muscle groups.[3] Although para-axial deep muscle groups probably play a relatively greater role in active postural stability, large multiple-joint muscle groups may also play a significant role in developing balance reactions because there may be greater proprioceptive feedback from a larger muscle mass.[3]

DEVELOPMENT OF POSTURAL CONTROL IN THE PRESENCE OF TORTICOLLIS

Congenital absence, denervation or abnormal coordination of specific muscle groups, especially if involvement is unilateral, may dramatically influence the development of the postural control system. Conditions such as Erb's palsy or torticollis can alter the balanced base of support or the interaction between deep and superficial muscle groups. Dysfunction in muscles such as the sternocleidomastoid (SCM), which may work as neck flexor, extensor, lateral flexor or rotator, depending on the orientation of its origin and insertion relative to the force of gravity and activation status of other muscles,[3] can have global implications for development of postural control.

Characteristics of Torticollis in the Supine Position

Infants with torticollis which does not significantly improve with early parental handling, repositioning and gentle stretching by three to four months of age are unable to center the head in midline alignment or move into a position of active chin tuck or capital flexion. They continue to have a strong sensory and postural bias toward neck and upper body asymmetry (see Figure 1, all Figures cited are in the Appendix). The head is held in lateral sidebend that varies in the amount of lateral neck flexion and a favored side of rotation. The most typical posture incorporates the movement components of unilateral SCM muscle contraction, combining rotation of the head to the contralateral side, lateral flexion ipsilaterally, and neck extension.[3] The infant is unable to actively position the head in midline alignment or turn to assume the opposite position of neck rotation and lateral flexion in supine, prone, supported sitting or supported standing. The characteristic posture includes shoulder hiking on the shortened side which varies with the degree of neck rotation. When neck rotation is less prominent, lateral side bend and shoulder hiking may be greater because the underlying stabilization of supportive postural muscle activity is lacking. Likewise, when neck rotation is a prominent component of posture or movement, lateral side bend and shoulder hiking may decrease because the greater neck rotation temporarily assists functional upper body stability.

Vision and Posture

Visual gaze is often oriented toward the side of head turning. This may be a direct result of biased perceptual sensorimotor experience resulting from visual access only to one side and the early postural connection between eye and head control in young infants.[1] With respect to this view of motor skill acquisition, head turning may be reinforced by visual interest as well.[5] For example, the infant in Figure 1, who was first seen for therapy at almost 4 months of age, retained persistent strong head turning to the left, despite her mother's attempts to reposition and encourage use of a greater variety of head positions. The mother's awareness of her infant's difficulties was intensified by the fact that her twin was available for direct comparison. Her mother recalls that social interaction with her infant with torticollis was frustrated by her sense that the child was disinterested in interaction and in the overall environment as compared to her twin sister. The infant's inability to stabilize and position her head interfered with her active engagement in social interaction.

This infant and other similar children have responded positively to gentle blocking of the visual field at the side of head turning preference resulting in improved visual engagement, fixation, and tracking, and even active head turning in the opposite direction. This simple strategy is easily applied by parents while using their face and vocal interaction as stimuli to maintain a young baby's motivation and interest. This same infant girl, who usually lay for extended periods unable to bring her hands together over her body, immediately became socially engaged, brought her hands together in midline and actively rubbed her feet together when her head and shoulders were cradled in a midline alignment with gentle neck traction. Slightly greater traction was applied on the shortened right side to encourage symmetry. Why did this head-centered position make such an immediate and dramatic difference in her movement control throughout the body? Did gently stabilizing the head in an age-appropriate position allow her to activate a central pattern generator that permitted a much different movement synergy to emerge?[6] Or was some mechanical change responsible? The mechanism remains to be discovered. The intriguing fact remains that gentle stabilization and positioning of the head in the posture characteristic of her age allowed an entirely different active sensorimotor experience to occur.

Characteristics of Torticollis in Prone Position

The typical fairly symmetrical and stable posture in the prone position at 3 to 4 months of age is also altered in infants with torticollis. Forearm weight bearing and head and upper body extension in prone are usually affected in these infants and more weight is distributed over the arm, trunk and pelvis on the affected side. Lateral neck flexion and shoulder hiking are pronounced on the affected side. These early patterns predispose the infant to asymmetry in later-appearing skills, such as weight shifting, reaching in prone, and sitting, and contribute to continued difficulties with head centering, trunk stability and balance.

Body Image

Tscharnuter described typical movement and balance organization of normally developing infants in terms of precise, active loading into support surfaces to stabilize and enable antigravity postural control and balance.[2] Early phases of postural control development are characterized by the need for a large area of contact with the surface. The area of contact narrows and becomes more precisely controlled as active proximal stability and balanced eccentric muscle control develop.[2] Deep pressure feedback from increasingly precise surface contacts is integrated with proprioceptive input from specific synergist muscle activation and from joint movements and other sensory inputs to develop an internal body map. This neural representation of the body includes the relationship between the location of the center of mass and the nature of the support surface.[6]

As compared to the typically developing 3- to 4-month-old infant, the infant with residual torticollis shows significantly altered postural control and, most likely, a significantly altered internal neural map or sensory body image (SBI) as well. The typical infant's postural control and internal body representation is characterized by strong symmetrical limb coordination, midline orientation with relatively symmetrical active loading into a broad surface of support and a centered head tending to return to midpositions following slight weightshifts.[1] In the typically developing infant of 3 to 4 months, midline visual interest and fixation, as well as repetitive symmetric motor activities reinforce a specific postural SBI.

The infant with torticollis, with a different sensorimotor experience probably has a significantly different postural SBI, which, nevertheless, is perceived by the infant as being "normal." Forceful alterations of their habitual body position and experience might be perceived as highly intrusive. Infants with torticollis may present with hypersensitivity to touch, deep pressure, and movement. They can be easily over-stimulated by visual, auditory and other typical sensory inputs. They often cry vigorously when stretch or deep pressure (as part of typical therapy techniques) is applied to tight neck, trunk and shoulder girdle areas. When viewed from the perspective of an altered SBI and significant difficulty in establishing appropriate postural sets for functional activity, this irritability and hypersensitivity makes sense.

Visual field manipulation and visual enticements, combined with active, gently assisted movement toward midline orientation, generally receives a more positive reaction from the infant than forceful stretch, although the response is often hesitant or puzzled as well. By using the technique mentioned earlier, blocking the visual field to the side of habitual head turning and engaging visual interest slowly from midline toward the opposite side, 3- to 4-month-old-infants with persistent torticollis are able to make relatively quick gains in active head turning in the supine position. Active head centering with chin tuck, which has a crucial connection to symmetrical shoulder, trunk, pelvis, and hip postural activity, seems more difficult to achieve. The reason for this may be the complexity involved in combining balanced deep muscle activation with more superficial neck muscle control as a foundation for these movements.[3] As an alternative explanation, imposition of a foreign experience on the infant with an altered SBI may make the combination of symmetrical and sustained head, shoulder, and trunk muscle activation especially difficult to achieve and sustain.

Effects of Poor Orientation to Midline

In the typically developing 3- to 4-month-old-infant, head centering, arm and leg lifting, downward visual gaze, and chin tuck in the supine position are associated with increased abdominal activation. As mentioned before, this combination is a predominant postural set reinforced over and over again by movement, fixation of visual gaze, and increasing sensory interest in hands and other body parts. Infants with torticollis have less abdominal muscle activation than is typical, especially during postural stabilizing functions and midline control. One could again speculate that poor development of this postural synergy is related to difficulty with head centering. General body stabilization for functional activity is, therefore, compromised.

Poor abdominal muscle activity in infants with torticollis has an impact on early sensorimotor development, diminishing active shoulder, trunk, pelvic, and hip stability necessary for graded righting and balance reactions, especially during backward weight shifting in sitting[6] and when making transitional movements from one position to another. One could speculate that they have a faulty SBI with an altered perception of the center of mass and a poor perceptual recognition of the nature of the support surface.[6]

An alternative hypothesis suggests that muscle mechanics are altered in the presence of torticollis. The oblique abdominal muscles act as rib stabilizers to assist shoulder girdle and arm stability and function. Shoulder girdle muscles taking their origins from the rib cage require a stable base in order to function normally. The shoulder girdle and rib cage complex, as the insertion point for many major neck muscle groups, including the clavicular portions of the SCM muscle, both contributes to and is affected by poorly coordinated neck muscular activity.[3]

Emphasis in therapy on abdominal muscle activity in sitting appears to be helpful for improving midline head orientation and active neck stabilization (Figure 2a). Precise weighting applied to the pelvis, the use of visual gaze to promote capital neck flexion and the use of a mobile surface, such as a gymnastic ball, which allows fine increments of motion and compression to facilitate ventral muscle activation, all seem to be helpful (Figure 2 a, b, c, d). Even after the infant is independently sitting, forward head control in midline frequently remains incomplete (Figure 2b). Persistence with therapy and home exercise to produce appropriate responses to backward displacement in sitting[6] appears to promote similar generalized trunk responses to backwards displacement in standing and walking at a later point in development. Abdominal and anterior neck muscle activation is a central feature of these postural responses.

Sternocleidomastoid Hypoextensibility

Another major impact of torticollis on the development of postural control, balance and movement results from persistent shortening of the affected SCM. This residual of SCM injury often appears as a persistent lateral neck flexion toward the affected side. The positional and movement components of this abnormal posture can be complex and may include shoulder elevation, lateral head tilt, and neck extension or rotation. Shortening on one side of the body produces an elongation of muscle groups on the other side. In addition to the altered SBI in which the asymmetrical position feels normal to the individual, muscle groups on the mechanically shortened side are hypothesized to generate more force in their shortened range. Those on the opposite elongated side are biomechanically at a disadvantage for strength of contraction.

Trunk and Extremity Reactions

Trunk elongation in righting and balance reactions is also directly related to changes in neck position. The infant quickly learns that one side "works better" than the other in the frontal plane. Balance responses and movement transitions which require weight shift from one side to the other or simultaneous activity of both sides are negatively affected by the neck asymmetry and lack of a stable head and neck posture. Movements affected include prone weight bearing and balance, pivot prone, rolling, active sitting balance, hands and knees activities, coming to sit with trunk rotation, and protective extension and limb loading reactions of the arms. The infant either moves so that the trunk always remains shortened on one side and lengthened on the other or finds a way to avoid the situation. In either case the postural base and resulting experience differs from that of the typical infant. Sequelae can be seen in older infants in their asymmetrical abilities and a general difficulty in achieving postural stability for balance reactions requiring double-arm support (Figures 3a, b, c, 4a). Protective extension reactions and movements requiring single-arm support are delayed and have poor quality (Figures 3d, e, 4b, c). For example, in responses to displacements in the frontal plane, the relative ease of lateral neck flexion on the affected side supports better arm support and leg reactions, but the arm on the affected side tends to adduct with elbow flexion instead of abducting to counterbalance the reaction on the opposite side (Figure 3d). The relative difficulty of achieving lateral neck flexion toward the unaffected side when lateral displacement occurs toward the side of the affected SCM creates a different compensatory pattern. For example, the child shown in Figure 3e with a shortened SCM on the right side has difficulty with lateral flexion toward the left. When she attempts to support on the right arm, she compensates for the lack of trunk elongation on the right side with a compensatory rotation of the body toward the weight-bearing arm, head rotation toward the left, left shoulder elevation and medial rotation of the left leg (Figure 3e). At 14 months, the same child has protective extension reactions which are more predictable and secure (Figure 4a). Independent upright mobility has developed, but some neck asymmetry is still noted. Limb reactions in response to lateral displacements are more bilaterally symmetrical (Figures 4b, c) and there is less need to compensate with left head turning. Left foot supination and left arm adduction against the trunk when she is displaced toward the right remain as persisting indicators of asymmetry (Figure 4c). Oblique lateral suspension at 14 months of age (Figures 4d, e) reveals some remaining difficulties with proximal stability, but strategies used include active neck flexion (Figure 4e) rather than body or head turning.

THERAPEUTIC INTERVENTION

Because of the implications of asymmetrical neck position on the development of postural control, balance and stability strategies, in this infant and others with persistent torticollis we focus our therapeutic intervention on vigorous oblique abdominal muscle activation (Figures 2a, b, c, d, 3a, b, c), the use of visual gaze to orient postural alignment (Figures 2c, d, 3b), deliberately planned limb loading on selected surfaces (Figures 2a, b, c, d, 3a, b, c, d, e, 4a, b, c), and gentle active movement to create displacements of the center of mass to evoke synergies combining neck, shoulder, trunk, and hip components in control of balance and posture. Because these infants would choose to master certain skills only in a single direction, we persist in using manual assists to evoke movements in the opposite direction even though it may be extremely difficult. In our experiences with using this combined sensorimotor approach, we find that infants are less irritable than with a more traditional stretching approach. Improvements in active neck range of motion and strength appear to be as good or better than with traditional stretching. Infants quickly gain range and control in neck rotation, but have more persistent difficulties with lateral head tilt and use of graded control in centering the head along the midline of the trunk. Rotational control, lateral neck muscle shortening and lack of head centering, tend to re-emerge as problems when the infant develops advanced postural sets, i.e., with initiation of sitting and crawling, standing, and walking. Specific help is needed with limb loading and stabilizing strategies when this happens. Continued active work is done by therapists and parents to maintain abdominal muscle strength and control for balance reactions and transitional movements, with emphasis on backward weight shift, graded control of diagonal movements, and refined symmetry of postural activation. Infants are generally discharged from therapy between 15 and 18 months of age when they show stable upright walking, stopping and turning with no obvious head and neck posture or weight transfer asymmetry. Parents are encouraged to continue active work on oblique abdominal muscles (play bouncing and "horse rides" on lap or therapy ball) and asked to check in with the therapist when the child begins to run or if head tilt or shoulder elevation should re-emerge.

CONCLUSION

Although individual differences in use of compensatory strategies may vary from child to child, infants with torticollis typically have decreased neck, shoulder, trunk, pelvic, and hip stability in midline orientation. This appears to be related to their altered early SBI and sensorimotor experience. A preference for asymmetrical weight bearing biases their postural stability, balancing reactions, and mechanics of muscles and joints. Functional skills tend to be developed which use these asymmetries and additional compensations while continuing to compromise maturation of graded midline postural control. By attempting to understand the interaction between isolated SCM injury and dysfunction and developing postural control and balance, and by implementing therapeutic intervention as described earlier, we hope to help children with persistent torticollis achieve a long lasting, efficient and flexible system for postural control and stability.

REFERENCES

1. Bly L. *Motor Skills Acquisition in the First Year of Life.* Tucson, AZ: Therapy Skill Builders; 1994.

2. Tscharnuter I. A new therapy approach to movement organization. *Physical & Occupational Therapy in Pediatrics.* 1993; 13(2):19-40.

3. Kapandji IA. *The Physiology of the Joints, Volume Three. The Trunk and Vertebral Column.* New York, NY: Churchill Livingstone; 1974.

4. Cioni G, Prechtl HFR. Preterm and early postterm motor behavior in low-risk premature infants. *Early Hum Dev.* 1990; 23:159-191.

5. Cech D, Martin S. *Functional Movement Development Across the Life Span.* Philadelphia, PA: WB Saunders Company; 1995.

6. Hirschfeld H, Forssberg H. Epigenetic development of postural responses for sitting during infancy. *Exp Brain Res.* 1994; 97:528-540.

APPENDIX

FIGURE 1. Felicia, Twin A, on the left at 2.5 months, shows the asymmetrical posture typical of torticollis with right SCM shortening.

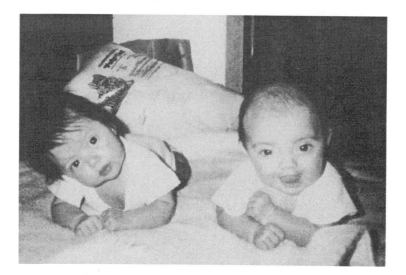

APPENDIX (continued)

FIGURE 2a. Treatment at 9 months of age uses pelvic stabilization into the gymnastic ball surface with slight backward displacement to assist ventral muscle activation.

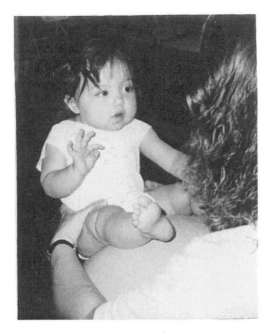

FIGURE 2b. She is unable to activate chin tuck, capital flexion and ventral postural muscle activity (abdominals and hip flexion for body righting), and shoulder elevation is seen as an attempt to compensate.

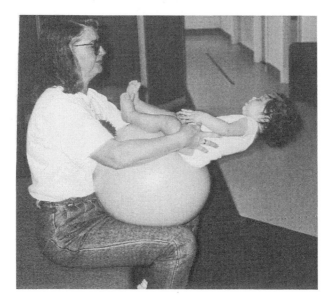

APPENDIX (continued)

FIGURE 2c. Visual fixation on her feet and on the therapist's face is used to assist chin tuck; ventral postural muscle activity improves and hands are free to play.

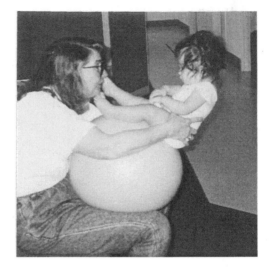

FIGURE 2d. Visual focus on a toy between the child's legs promotes a forward head position and ventral postural muscle activity. The therapist's manual contacts are brought distally to the knees with active loading into the ball surface and with backward displacement. Small bounces are used to assist sustained ventral postural muscle activity and provide proprioceptive input.

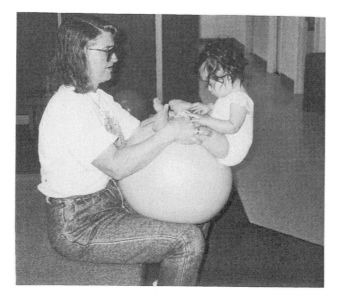

APPENDIX (continued)

FIGURE 3a. At 12 months, Felicia has incomplete forward protective extension of the arms which compromises her willingness to risk falling in the
upright position and delays the development of independent standing and
walking.

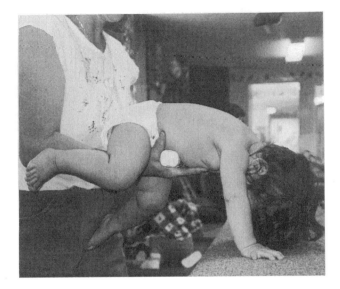

FIGURE 3b. Visual fixation elicited between the legs assists chin tuck, neck elongation and upper body stability in an inverted weight bearing position. Her insecurity with forward weight shift onto her arms is seen in a backward weight shift of her pelvis, ankle plantar flexion, and toe curling.

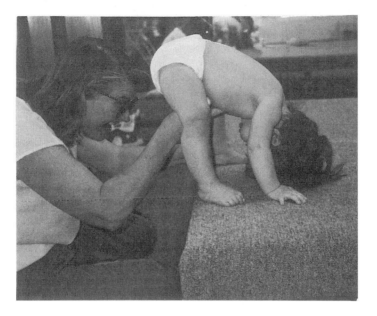

APPENDIX (continued)

FIGURE 3c. At 12 months, generation of stable balance from hand and foot surface contact is difficult, as noted by neck hyperextension and poor activation of oblique abdominal muscles. In bear-walk position, active balance on hands and feet is assisted with abdominal support and activation. This important transitional position is typically used to maneuver through free squat to stand and to climb over low obstacles. The increased neck hyperextension indicates decreased postural stabilization in upper body.

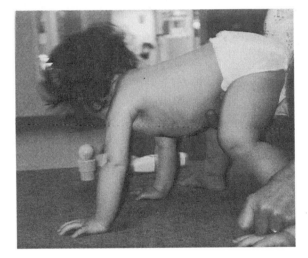

FIGURE 3d. Active weight support on the left arm is facilitated by right lateral neck flexion. Her right arm remains adducted against her side showing a decreased base of postural stability.

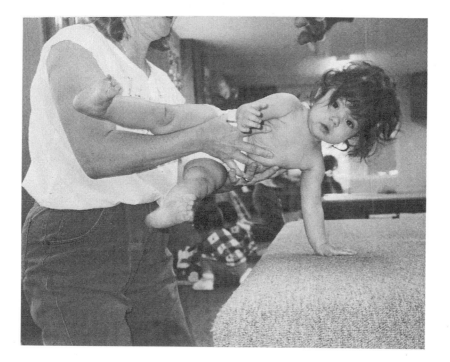

APPENDIX (continued)

FIGURE 3e. As compared with Figure 3d, active weight support on the right arm is difficult because of poor left lateral neck muscle activation. Head turning to the left, body turning toward the right arm, left shoulder hiking, left leg internal rotation and foot supination are all believed to be compensatory maneuvers resulting from decreased postural stability.

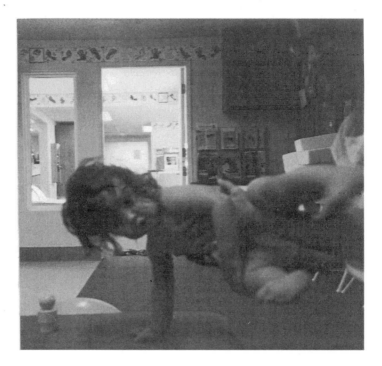

FIGURE 4a. At 14 months, Felicia has more stable forward weight bearing on arms as indicated by improved active midrange neck extension. Her feet engage each other to support the activity because of inadequate central axis stability.

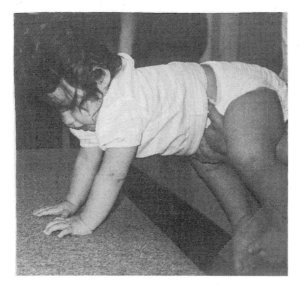

APPENDIX (continued)

FIGURE 4b. Active weight bearing on left arm now shows relatively full development of postural reactions in arms and legs.

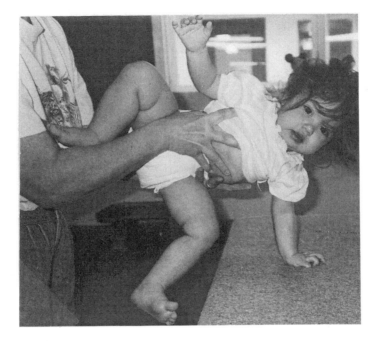

FIGURE 4c. Decreased left lateral neck flexion is still seen, although it is much improved. Better neck muscle activation supports improved postural organization, allowing better quality active weight bearing over the right hand. As compared with Figure 3e, there are fewer body and limb compensatory reactions although the left shoulder adduction and foot supination remain as signals of continued postural organization difficulties.

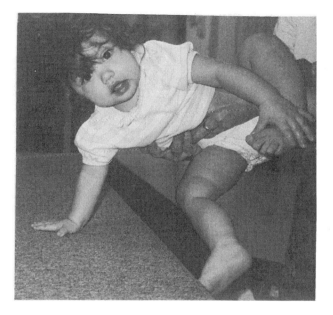

APPENDIX (continued)

FIGURE 4d. The oblique balancing response in the air is relatively complete with active full elongation of the downward (left) side, supporting graded shortening of the upward (right) side. Grabbing on with the right hand indicates a certain degree of remaining postural instability. Slight left head turning or increased right lateral neck flexion or shoulder hiking are often seen in challenging new situations.

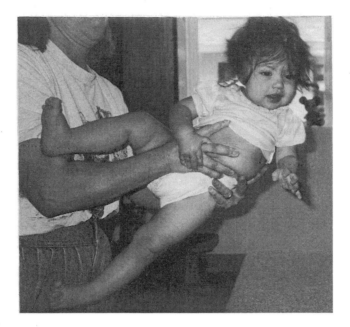

FIGURE 4e. The oblique balancing response still shows increased difficulties with generation of full postural responses on the left side although neck
flexion has now replaced the earlier more asymmetrical compensations
shown in Figure 3e. Shoulder and trunk activity mirrors that of the neck with
more symmetrical increased ventral activity. The right side active elongation
response and left side graded shortening response are decreased relative
to Figure 4d and also influence her limb responses.

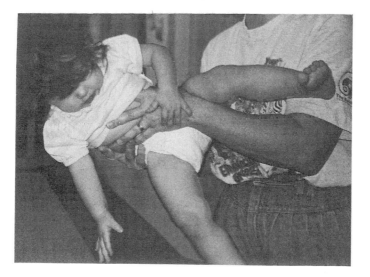

Epilogue

Over the past 11 years of clinical practice, I have spent countless hours documenting clinical findings in children with torticollis using a variety of methods. It became a singular quest for me to understand how to assess and evaluate findings in order to provide appropriate treatment for torticollis. Hours have been spent searching the literature to find explanations for what I was observing and documenting as a clinician. Three features typically studied and reported in the literature are range of neck muscle motion, persistence of head tilt, and facial symmetry.

I believe that there are more questions to be asked and more answers to find. Future research is needed to answer these questions:

1. At what rate do infants and children gain or regain strength in muscle groups that are contractured or have disuse atrophy?
2. What is the rate of spontaneous recovery without conservative intervention versus the rate of recovery with conservative intervention?
3. At what rate do postural reactions develop and muscle activation patterns and timing sequences return in infants and children who have congenital asymmetries of range of motion and strength?
4. How does home program and therapy affect rate of recovery?
5. What are the typical movement patterns and motor skill deficits of children with torticollis?
6. Is there a difference in attainment of motor skill development in infants and children who have the initial asymmetries of

[Haworth co-indexing entry note]: "Epilogue." Co-published simultaneously in *Physical & Occupational Therapy in Pediatrics* (The Haworth Press, Inc.) Vol. 17, No. 2, 1997, pp. 119-120; and: *Torticollis: Differential Diagnosis, Assessment and Treatment, Surgical Management and Bracing* (ed: Karen Karmel-Ross) The Haworth Press, Inc., 1997, pp. 119-120. Single or multiple copies of this article are available for a fee from The Haworth Document Delivery Service [1-800-342-9678, 9:00 a.m. - 5:00 p.m. (EST). E-mail address: getinfo@haworth.com].

119

range of motion and strength associated with a torticollis posture?

7. What role does underlying postural tone and neuromuscular coordination play in the recovery rate of infants and children with torticollis?

8. How is variety in motor response affected by the limited neck and trunk movement in infants and children with torticollis?

9. What possible role does a deficit in central vestibular connections have to the activation response in an overstretched SCM muscle?

10. What role does range of motion and strength play in the ability to adapt postural muscle responses to changes in position?

11. What are the typical postural muscle synergies of infants and children with torticollis posture?

12. Do patients with persistent head tilt develop abnormal visual perception as a compensatory mechanism for asymmetrical head posture?

13. Why does a preference posture persist in the infant and child with torticollis?

The improved functional outcome of answering these clinical questions may come from new insights into the pathomechanics associated with torticollis posture, the developmental characteristics of congenital muscular torticollis, and the strategic building blocks for planning and sequencing intervention for children with torticollis.

In closing, I thank the people who were supportive and helped me to continue my quest during the times I felt like abandoning it. You know who you are . . . thank you all.

Karen Karmel-Ross

Index

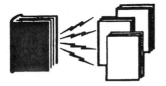

Haworth
DOCUMENT DELIVERY
SERVICE

This valuable service provides a single-article order form for any article from a Haworth journal.

- *Time Saving:* No running around from library to library to find a specific article.
- *Cost Effective:* All costs are kept down to a minimum.
- *Fast Delivery:* Choose from several options, including same-day FAX.
- *No Copyright Hassles:* You will be supplied by the original publisher.
- *Easy Payment:* Choose from several easy payment methods.

Open Accounts Welcome for . . .
- Library Interlibrary Loan Departments
- Library Network/Consortia Wishing to Provide Single-Article Services
- Indexing/Abstracting Services with Single Article Provision Services
- Document Provision Brokers and Freelance Information Service Providers

---

MAIL or *FAX* THIS ENTIRE ORDER FORM TO:

Haworth Document Delivery Service
The Haworth Press, Inc.
10 Alice Street
Binghamton, NY 13904-1580

or FAX: 1-800-895-0582
or CALL: 1-800-342-9678
9am-5pm EST

PLEASE SEND ME PHOTOCOPIES OF THE FOLLOWING SINGLE ARTICLES:
1) Journal Title: _____

    Vol/Issue/Year: _____ Starting & Ending Pages: _____

Article Title: _____

2) Journal Title: _____

    Vol/Issue/Year: _____ Starting & Ending Pages: _____

Article Title: _____

3) Journal Title: _____

    Vol/Issue/Year: _____ Starting & Ending Pages: _____

Article Title: _____

4) Journal Title: _____

    Vol/Issue/Year: _____ Starting & Ending Pages: _____

Article Title: _____

(See other side for Costs and Payment Information)

COSTS: Please figure your cost to order quality copies of an article.

1. Set-up charge per article: $8.00

        ($8.00 × number of separate articles)   _____

2. Photocopying charge for each article:

                    1-10 pages: $1.00   _____

                    11-19 pages: $3.00   _____

                    20-29 pages: $5.00   _____

                    30+ pages: $2.00/10 pages   _____

3. Flexicover (optional): $2.00/article   _____

4. Postage & Handling: US: $1.00 for the first article/

                    $.50 each additional article   _____

                    Federal Express: $25.00   _____

                    Outside US: $2.00 for first article/

                    $.50 each additional article_____

5. Same-day FAX service: $.35 per page   _____

                            GRAND TOTAL: _____

METHOD OF PAYMENT: (please check one)

❑ Check enclosed   ❑ Please ship and bill. PO # _____

                  (sorry we can ship and bill to bookstores only! All others must pre-pay)

❑ Charge to my credit card: ❑ Visa; ❑ MasterCard; ❑ Discover;

                  ❑ American Express;

Account Number:_____ Expiration date:_____

Signature: ✗_____

Name: _____ Institution: _____

Address: _____

_____

City: _____ State:_____ Zip:_____

Phone Number: _____ FAX Number: _____

MAIL or *FAX* THIS ENTIRE ORDER FORM TO:

Haworth Document Delivery Service | **or FAX:** 1-800-895-0582
The Haworth Press, Inc. | **or CALL:** 1-800-342-9678
10 Alice Street | 9am-5pm EST)
Binghamton, NY 13904-1580